João Paulo Guimarães (ed.)
Fear of Aging

Contemporary Literature | Volume 15

João Paulo Guimarães holds a PhD in English from SUNY Buffalo, was an Irish Research Council postdoctoral fellow at University College Dublin and is currently a junior researcher at the Universidade do Porto. His research concentrates on experimental poetry and science studies.

João Paulo Guimarães (ed.)
Fear of Aging
Old Age in Horror Fiction and Film

[transcript]

This collection was edited as part of research developed at the Comparative Literature Institute Margarida Losa, an R & D Unit financed by the Portuguese government via FCT – Fundação para a Ciência e a Tecnologia (UIDB/00500/2020 – https ://doi.org/10.54499/UIDB/00500/2020). An electronic version of this book is freely available, thanks to the support of libraries working with Knowledge Unlatched. KU is a collaborative initiative designed to make high quality books Open Access for the public good. The Open Access ISBN for this book is 978-3-8394-6195-2. More information about the initiative and links to the Open Access version can be found at w ww.knowledgeunlatched.org.

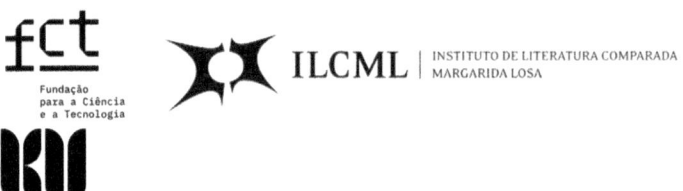

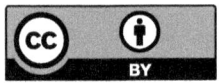

Bibliographic information published by the Deutsche Nationalbibliothek
The Deutsche Nationalbibliothek lists this publication in the Deutsche Nationalbibliografie; detailed bibliographic data are available in the Internet at https://dnb.dnb.de/

This work is licensed under the Creative Commons Attribution 4.0 (BY) license, which means that the text may be remixed, transformed and built upon and be copied and redistributed in any medium or format even commercially, provided credit is given to the author. Creative Commons license terms for re-use do not apply to any content (such as graphs, figures, photos, excerpts, etc.) not original to the Open Access publication and further permission may be required from the rights holder. The obligation to research and clear permission lies solely with the party re-using the material.

First published in 2024 by transcript Verlag, Bielefeld
© João Paulo Guimarães (Ed.)

transcript Verlag | Hermannstraße 26 | D-33602 Bielefeld | live@transcript-verlag.de

Cover layout: Maria Arndt, Bielefeld
Cover illustration: Sofia Matos Silva
Printed by: Majuskel Medienproduktion GmbH, Wetzlar
https://doi.org/10.14361/9783839461952
Print-ISBN: 978-3-8376-6195-8 | PDF-ISBN: 978-3-8394-6195-2
ISSN of series: 2701-9470 | eISSN of series: 2703-0474

Printed on permanent acid-free text paper.

Contents

Introduction
Old Monsters and the Monsters of Old 7

"Grateful for the Time We Have Been Given"
Cinematic Aging in the Films of M. Night Shyamalan
Michael J. Blouin 9

A Horrifying Reversal
The Dislocating Impact of Age Consciousness in "The Curious Case of Benjamin Button"
Michael S. D. Hooper 23

There's No Cure
Failures of the Aged under Neoliberalism
Kaydee Corbin Anderson and Ahoo Tabatabai 45

The Southern Slasher Comes of Age
Old Age, Race, and Disability in Ti West's *X*
Rose Steptoe 63

"With Strange Aeons Even Death May Die"
Aging in the World of Cthulhu
Joel Soares Oliveira 79

"And I'm Going to Get Old"
Age Horror in the *Twilight* Franchise
Ruth Gehrmann 93

Claudia: The Forever Child and Vampire Killer in Anne Rice's
Interview with the Vampire
Kimberly Smith 111

Childhood at the Center
The Horror of Miles and Flora in Henry James's *The Turn of the Screw*
(1898) and Jack Clayton's Film Adaptation *The Innocents* (1961)
Vitor Alves Silva 129

Old Age and Disability as Alterity
Ghosts, (Constructions of) Normalcy and Reliability in *The Others*
Mariana Castelli-Rosa 153

Fears of Old Age, Cultural Representations of Elders and
Narrative Twists of Aging in Four Horror Episodes of the *Twilight Zone*
Marta Miquel-Baldellou 169

Uncanny Female Aging in Dahl's Horror
Ieva Stončikaitė 201

Two Witches at the School
Aging and Instruction in Argento's and Guadagnino's *Suspiria* Films
André Assis Almeida and João Paulo Guimarães 217

Alzheimer's Disease as Demonic Possession in Adam Robitel's
The Taking of Deborah Logan **(2014)**
Elisabete Lopes 229

Beyond the Horror of the Aging Female
Decay, Regeneration and *Relic* (Natalie Erika James, 2020)
Laura Hubner 247

Introduction
Old Monsters and the Monsters of Old

In her 2017 book *Forgotten*, Marlene Goldman notes that the media often adopts a Gothic
register and use apocalyptic language to describe the rise in dementia cases across the west in recent decades. The disease is figured as a "silent killer" that threatens to erase our identities, turning us and our loved ones into a faceless zombie mob. But horror is a genre that is often deployed to depict old people more generally, not just those debilitated by disease. One has only
to think of the witches that populate cultural texts of all sorts, from *Macbeth* and "Snow White" to *Game of Thrones*. In such instances, horror is used to evoke not just a fear of death but a fear of aging, older age being equated with bodily, mental and social decline.

On the other hand, the idea of the unnatural extension of the lifespan has also generated its own brand of horror. Immortality may be something humans, at least since the time of *Gilgamesh*, have always sought to attain, but its pursuit has invariably entailed some sort of retribution. For vampires, eternal life is a curse that forces them to feed on the blood of the young to maintain their decrepit existence (a trope that is eerily evocative of the unfortunate stereotype of the present-day pensioner). Movies like Terry Gilliam's Brazil (which highlights the risks and implications of plastic surgery) also express the reservations many have about the powers of technology to unnaturally prolong youth.

Recent and more subversive takes on the genre might be especially productive for our discussion about aging and older age. Novels like *The*

Girl with All the Gifts or *Handling the Undead*, for example, ask us to rethink the figure of the zombie and how we might relate to such creatures were we ever to be irreversibly overrun by them. Would we be able to coexist with zombies, say, if they posed no imminent danger to us? A question very much like this is posed by the film *Relic*, which is at the center of a few of essays in this collection. Like *Relic*, the novel *White Is for Witching* foregrounds intergenerational bonds, the monster it revolves around being a *soucouyant*, a witch/ghost that is repellant not so much because she is old but rather because it congregates it herself the bodies of women from three different generations.

In this book we investigate what exactly we are afraid of when we posit old age as a source of horror. We will examine the different kinds of fear associated with aging and assess if and how these fears can be allayed. The essays in this collection grapple with such topics as: the fear of backwardness, conservatism and irrationality (which we often unfairly associate with people that live in rural areas or with little education); aging backwards and children that behave like adults; fear of losing one's memory and identity; the persistence of the past in the present (haunts, curses and ghosts); fear of disability and dependence. As Leo Braudy reminds us in *Haunted*, fear is historical. As such, it can be interrogated, debunked and perhaps dispelled. Our ultimate aim is to harness the thrills and pleasures of horror to think about how quality of life can be improved in old age and how older people can be better integrated in our ever fearful and suspicious societies.

"Grateful for the Time We Have Been Given"
Cinematic Aging in the Films of M. Night Shyamalan

Michael J. Blouin[1]

Filmmaker M. Night Shyamalan habitually uses cinematic structure to convey larger thematic concerns. Consider, for example, the ways that his 2006 film *Lady in the Water* plays with audience expectations to comment upon the nature of modern storytelling.[2] In that vein, Shyamalan's recent work turns to the question of aging in order to reflect upon the relationship between filmmaker and film-goer. Two of his horror films, *The Visit* (2015) and *Old* (2021), inspire anxieties about getting older and, at the same time, reveal how cinematic form can alleviate those very fears.

Originally titled *Sundowning*, Shyamalan's *The Visit* conveys the palpable terror of an elderly couple suffering from ill health and the subsequent unease of their young wards. It exposes how audiences approach a film with certain expectations, or plans, in mind; however, what Shyamalan's audiences receive never matches the initial blueprint. The form as well as the content of *The Visit* forces spectators to contrast their initial sense of mastery, which is to say, their belief that they can know what is coming, with the unexpected events that actually unfold. The uneasy wards make a documentary about their aging caretakers. As they piece together important bits of the footage, audience members

---

1 Milligan University.
2 Patrick Collier argues, Shyamalan routinely comments upon his own "narratological structure" (Collier 2008: 270). *The Village*, for instance, is a "narrative that self-consciously foregrounds and exaggerates its own manipulations" (270).

confront the distinction between the *fabula* (the chronology of the story) and the *syuzhet* (the ordering of the story by the editor). In turn, what initially appears to be unnerving – "sundowning," a term that describes the effects of dementia – reveals itself to be a sort of gift: the ability to accept cinema as it is, in the present, without preconditions. In this way, Shyamalan offers a corrective to contemporary film consumption through his sustained reflection upon the aging process.

Shyamalan's *Old* likewise reflects upon getting older as a uniquely cinematic experience (and vice versa). A group of unwitting tourists are lured onto a mysterious beach that rapidly ages them. Over the span of the film, movie-goers watch as the physical and mental states of the characters deteriorate. Shyamalan again places the spectator in an uncomfortable position: like the cold, clinical scientists that observe this traumatic event from atop nearby ridgelines, the spectator must gaze upon the innocent characters as they struggle to make sense of what is happening to them. The life of any fictional character is always already confined to the life span of a given narrative, and so Shyamalan presents parallels between the accelerated aging that takes place within the framework of a cinematic story and the illusion of plentiful time that enables most human beings to recognize the joys of aging only at the dusk of their days, when Minerva's owl at long last takes flight. In sum, Shyamalan's horror films *The Visit* and *Old* contemplate the fears of aging through meta-commentaries upon cinematic structure.

As an auteur, Shyamalan habitually preoccupies himself with the idea that spectators ought to coexist with the cinematic experience in a less plotted way and concurrently learn how to age more gracefully.[3] Shyamalan's thrillers condition spectators to confront the uncertainties of the filmic experience as a corollary of aging. Do not fear the future, the film insists, or let the past weigh too heavily upon you – instead, enjoy the temporal flow, aesthetically as well as existentially.

---

3   The type of work done in this chapter looks to uncover, in the words of Geoffrey Nowell-Smith, "what gives an author's work its particular structure, both defining it internally and distinguishing one body of work from another" (qtd. in Wollen 2004: 567).

First, Shyamalan's recent films instigate living in the throes of time with an underlying confidence in a retrospective order to be imposed by the auteur's (in)famous twist endings. Second, these films ask the spectator to appreciate the fullness of cinematic moments – unedited; lived duration – as though they are a poetic gift: a romantic presentism that transcends the psychical confines of a skeptical age. Simply put, Shyamalan's working thesis is that cinema trains audiences to live in the moment.

Many of Shyamalan's films render literal the fear of aging by featuring characters that do not want to acknowledge their own mortality, from the ongoing denial of Malcolm Crowe (Bruce Willis) in *The Sixth Sense* (1999) to the desperate question posed by Edward Walker (William Hurt) in *The Village*: who will be left to safeguard the utopian community once the elders have perished? The two films considered at some length in this chapter (*The Visit* and *Old*) heighten this simmering sense of dread by shining a spotlight upon the painful ailments of their senior characters. At the same time, many of Shyamalan's films compel audiences to consider the temporal nature of the film-going experience. Although a given film can certainly play with time – consider, for instance, flashbacks, or the ability for a film's jump cuts to advance a story from one point in time to a distant point in the future – no editing trick can slow the relentless march of time. Nothing can stop the end of the film from coming. Shyamalan ostensibly focuses so much of his attention on surprise endings in part because he wants the spectator to be hyper-aware of this relentless march: the runaway sensation that undergirds the thriller genre. But alongside these acute feelings of dread, uncertainty, and relentlessness (primary feelings that accompany one's ever-advancing years), Shyamalan's films foster a blind faith in the cinematic flow – or, more specifically, in the cinematic flow of his own films, which appear to evade the acumen of audience members and defy strained efforts to anticipate the director's well-crafted plots. Find joy in the ride, these cinematic texts implore their audience. If Shyamalan's spectators accept this challenge, they can theoretically stop fearing old age.

Deep Moments

The Visit thoroughly establishes the concept of aging as an abject fear. One character observes, "People are scared of old people for no reason." From graphic displays of incontinence – when "Pop Pop" (Peter McRobbie) pushes the face of Tyler (Ed Oxenbould) into his soiled diapers – to the unsettling symptoms of dementia – when Nana (Deanna Dunagan) wields a knife and erratically wanders the house after 9:30 pm – Shyamalan's film amplifies the dread of getting older. The film concludes with an anxiety-inducing family game night in which, Pop Pop declares, "the young" must face off against "the old." During the final encounter, aspiring filmmaker Becca (Olivia DeJonge) encounters her Nana wrapped in a white sheet, donning the traditional garb of the costumed ghost, in a moment that highlights the closing act of the aging process, that is, death itself. Is Shyamalan an ageist because he depicts the elderly as objects of revulsion?

I would argue that *The Visit*, beneath its derivative stylization (it borrows heavily from popular found footage films like *The Blair Witch Project* or the *Paranormal Activity* series), is a thoughtful meditation on a latent link between the cinematic experience and the experience of aging. Like most of Shyamalan's thrillers, there is an uncertain future, a twist yet to come, and there is a disquieting past with which the characters must reckon in order to move on. As such, this film – like any film, really – pulls the spectator between what has happened previously and what still lies ahead. The audience watches as the aspiring filmmaker (Becca) constructs a linear narrative, with mounting tension and conventional beats. Simultaneously, though, Becca expresses a frustrated desire to evade such heavy-handed manipulation and swim instead in the waters of *cinéma vérité*. Early in the film, Becca commands Tyler to stop trying to make a swing move on its own: "Let it naturally swing." In a state of distress after showing her brother some of her naturalist footage, she asks him, "Are you consciously aware that that's my intention?" Becca wants to make a film that captures reality *as it is*, without her intervention, yet she keeps meeting strangers that consider themselves to be actors and mug for her camera. Given his own aspirations as a free-style rapper, Tyler too prefers simultaneity to plotted design. In a perverse sort of way, then, these two young artists have much to learn from the murderous couple posing as their grandparents, since the elderly duo has lost all sense of linear time: Pop Pop repeatedly thinks he is headed to a costume party from his past, and Nana goes through the motions of an earlier life.

Although classical Hollywood cinema uses editing tricks to manage the spectator's experience of time, cinema also has the capacity to glimpse "real time" in the unaltered roll of the camera. Against the confines of the clock, a correlation between the artificial ways that human beings plot their own lives into concrete units (hours, days, weeks, etc.) and the artificial ways that directors move spectators through a film's ninety-minute run time, *The Visit* posits a different kind of cinematic experience, one that simultaneously invites a different experience of aging. Just as Becca utilizes her camera to bash open a lock and escape from the house of horrors, and just as Becca considers her film to be an "elixir" to help her family heal from a recent painful divorce, Shyamalan appears to believe that cinema promises a new approach to being in time. He suggests this new approach in at least two ways: first, Becca's "perfect cinematic images," her interstitial shots, or caesuras, that capture a still moment without the baggage of a weighty past or a loaded future; second, a surprise ending that retroactively imposes a sense of comfort that neither character nor spectator need worry because the auteur will inevitably instill orderliness and so the parties involved should learn to enjoy the flow and simply stay in the moment. Age is a mere number; indulge in the cinematic present.

The interstitial shots in *The Visit* speak volumes. Sometimes the camera lingers on the sky as it transitions from day into night. At other times, the camera lingers on the moon, in seemingly impossible shots because Becca is not allowed outside of her room after 9:30 pm. In these quiet moments, the film quite literally calls to mind the philosopher Immanuel Kant's rumination on the starry skies above: is one's experience of time subjective or objective?[4] In one sense, these artful shots mark the subjective passage of time, as the film moves steadily from one day to the next, the duration of the torturous visit being stressed in bold font (Monday Morning, Tuesday Morning, and so forth). These symbolist inserts contribute to a subjective sense of time passing that Becca – and Shyamalan – meticulously constructs for the spectator. In another sense, though, these pregnant shots evoke the fullness of the cinematic image as a temporal experience: one unedited roll of Becca's camera, usually focused upon a natural phenomenon that it is itself a sign of eternity and/or the cycles that comprise a steady, and arguably more objective, perception of time. As the film itself "ages," and moves towards its preconceived *denoument*, the audience is asked to stop anticipating the contrivances of plot – the terrors of a thriller's cadence – and revel instead in the capacity of cinema to convey the poignant stillness of an enduring presentism.

Shyamalan appears to be preoccupied with this approach to cinematic presentism. *Lady in the Water*, for instance, ends with a shot of the protagonist (Paul Giamatti) gazing up at the starry sky as his ward, the story itself (embodied in a character played by Bryce Dallas Howard), flies away. As the rapidly aging avatar for the film's story reveals, the cinematic experience is frequently a contrived race against the clock. But it offers a type of elixir, too, in the form of shots that convey something much bigger and (arguably) more objective: namely, a sense of being in time uninterrupted by subjective editorializing. Or one might consider the final shot of Shyamalan's *The Village*: the injured hero (Joaquin Phoenix) awakens to see the members of his village standing around him, suddenly hopeful of the future. The spectator shares the hero's gaze and she is meant to share in his renewed optimism as well. Prior to this shot, the elder statesman of the village (William Hurt) has forfeited his capacity to control, literally and figuratively, the clocks of his sheltered community. He has given up his valuable antique pocket watch in exchange for a life-saving medicine from the modern world,

---

4   As David Couzens Hoy writes, "The reality of temporality seems equally objective and subjective" (Hoy 2012: xv).

beyond the gates of his self-fashioned utopia. The sense of being in time within the fictional village, as well as within the film *The Village*, is a tightly monitored affair. The past and the future are almost always kept in their "proper" place. When the elder statesman gives up his watch, and accepts the risks of exposing the past and opening up to an uncertain future, he at last holds true to a creed that he has uttered several times throughout the film: "We are grateful for the time we have been given." In the closing shot of *The Village*, the spectator again appreciates Becca's "perfect cinematic image": a transcendent, evocative image that exists in "real time," somehow inside yet outside of the overly-curated rhythms of the typical Hollywood thriller. Although one might try to arrange one's life in a neat-and-tidy temporal package, one with a clear beginning, middle, and end, Shyamalan argues that cinema can expose audiences to a way of being present in the here and now.

The Visit doubles down upon this concept by employing found footage of the murderous Nana as well as home videos of the neglectful father. When Becca elects to insert home videos of her father, it is both an act of forgiveness on her part and, at the same time, a Bergsonian reminder that the past, present, and future forever overlap with one another. These private videos remain the past as well as the future of *The Visit* – and, ultimately, they are supposed to be viewed as yet another example of a deeper cinematic present. This sense of a deeper cinematic present captures something organic that cannot be plotted in advance. These moments are designed to look spontaneous, and they prove to be the very *cinéma vérité* that Becca has been seeking all along. She (and the spectator) are instructed to overcome their fear of getting older, that is, of living a life that feels too scripted and reaches a contrived conclusion, by appreciating the profound presentism on display in the unfiltered cinematic object. These images of the world are, as film critic Andre Bazin argues, "formed automatically, without the creative intervention of man." Bazin famously contends that "cinema is objectivity in time… the image of [things in] their duration, change mummified" (Bazin 2004: 168–169). Of course, these profilmic, "natural" events are always-already part of Shyamalan's larger design, and so the spectator might reasonably counter that the film's presumed presentism is only ever just another illusion generated by the filmmaker.[5] Nonetheless, Shyamalan's found footage is meant to resolve the problem posed by excessive plotting.

The Visit inspires in its audience both a fear of aging and, concurrently, a faith in cinema's magical power to defeat death. "Time passing, duration, and change," Philip Rosen asserts, "are exactly what Bazin's ontological subject is driven to *disavow*, for they raise the problem of death" (Rosen 2001: 28, author's emphasis). By investing a great deal in deep moments, Bazin's imagined filmmaker strives to evade the haunting specter of aging and therefore exert "fantastic control" over the "causation of death" (23). Shyamalan and his mouthpiece Becca ask the spectator to endow the cinematic image with "an unprecedented credibility" and thus transcend her assumed anxieties about aging (23). That is to say, *The Visit* defeats its abject elderly subjects in the name of preserving cinema's capacity to defeat death, thereby re-enforcing Bazin's argument in regards to the central impetus of the cinematic medium.

Going with the Flow

At this point, let us turn to Shyamalan's signature move as an auteur: his unexpected plot twists. Since his inaugural film *The Sixth Sense*, Shyamalan has consistently quilted his films with unexpected endings that re-define everything that came before them. Such unexpected endings produce feelings of *uncertainty* in the audience about what is to come, and they also paradoxically produce feelings of *comfort* by promising that every event in the sequence of the film will eventually "make sense." To age alongside the unfolding of a Shyamalan film, then, is to confront the dread of endings, be they mortal or aesthetic. At the same time, the Shyamalan twist, which remains predictable that a spectator could set his watch to it, diffuses this dread by instilling in the story, retroactively,

---

5   Philip Rosen writes that cinema's ostensibly "fantastic defense against time" is in fact a construct: "There is something inevitably illusory in this apparently complete concreteness" (Rosen 2001: 21, 13).

a sense of order and purpose: "The active quest of the [spectator] for those shaping ends that, terminating the dynamic process of [viewing], promise to bestow meaning and significance on the beginning and the middle" (Brooks 1984: 19).[6] As Peter Brooks argues, "What remains to be [seen] will restructure the provisional meanings of the already [viewed]" (23). In Shyamalan's hands, a thriller's surprise ending doubles as a commentary about the experience of being in time: as the seemingly meaningless, random events that occur within a person's lifespan – or within the lifespan of a given narrative – invariably come together in a proper fashion, the character/spectator lets go of futile attempts to predict or plot the proceedings and instead focuses on enjoying the experience of the film, safe in the hands of a presumably loving auteur.

If my thesis proves correct, and one of Shyamalan's main preoccupations is the latent connection between the angst of aging and watching a film, then *Old* should be considered his crowning achievement. While films like *The Visit* gesture at this underlying schematic in a variety of ways, they do not directly link the running time of the film to the duration of a character's life. *Old*, on the other hand, makes this link quite literal: the spectator must watch as characters stranded on a mysterious beach grow older at an alarming rate. Indebted to Alfred Hitchcock, Shyamalan's films are metacommentaries about filmmaking and the voyeuristic pleasures as well as perversities of spectatorship. As a character in *Old* cries out, "Let's concentrate on the issue at hand: do you know about movies?" *Old* asks its audience to interrogate the fraught relationship between cinematic time and the various other ways in which characters/spectators might spend their precious remaining moments. An actuary (Gael Garcia Bernal) fights with his archivist partner (Vicky Krieps) over their conflicting attitudes about temporality: whereas the archivist accuses the actuary of obsessing over the future, the actuary

---

6 Frank Kermode adds, "[Men] need fictive concords with origins and ends, such as give meaning to lives and to poems. The End they imagine will reflect their irreducibly intermediary preoccupations. They fear it, and as far as we can see have always done so; the End is a figure for their own deaths (...) So, perhaps, are all ends in fiction" (Kermode 2000: 7).

accuses the archivist of clinging to the past (she only agrees to go to the mysterious beach because it will one day prove to be a "good memory" for her family). Meanwhile, Shyamalan makes familiar gestures at presentism: when the archivist interrupts the exuberant singing of her daughter in the back seat (Thomasin Mackenzie), her daughter berates her for stripping away the spontaneity of the moment; the actuary uncharacteristically saves his partner's life by making a "fast decision" to cut a rapidly growing tumor out of her belly; at the end of the film, the remaining characters wonder why they have been so obsessed with escaping from the beach – one character declares that "it's so beautiful" while the son of the actuary and archivist (Emmun Elliott) pauses during his escape from the beach to make a sand castle. A human life can feel a lot like a ninety-minute film in that the subject could feel compelled to either speed toward a redemptive ending or slow down the figurative runaway train. "Whatever is happening to us," a character complains, "is happening very fast." *Old* remains Shyamalan's most sustained attempt to date to condition its spectators to stop fearing old age and appreciate the present moment.

The spectator of *Old* remains both engrossed in the aging process and, concomitantly, estranged from it. To enter the experience of watching a film requires that an audience enter the flow of time as it has been generated by that particular film. Yet cinema also alienates spectators from their temporal norms by forcing them to reflect upon the artifice of man-made temporalities. On the one hand, "both in filming and projection, the cinema is a kind of clockwork mechanism, exposing and projecting immobile photograms at regular, equidistant intervals" (Lim 2009: 11). Through a plethora of techniques – parallelism, simultaneity, *leitmotifs*, and so forth – the filmmaker, like the elder statesman in *The Village*, "keeps time," in that he regulates the beats and cadences of the film-going situation. When a spectator walks out onto the mysterious beach alongside the characters in *Old*, she too must languish in the unique temporality of this suspenseful narrative. *Time grows ever shorter for characters and audience members alike.* On the other hand, cinema can "provoke a critical reassessment of modern time consciousness" (ibid: 11). After all, Shyamalan's spectator is never fully a part of the tribe on the beach – she stands at the perimeter, watching, not unlike the scientists that stalk along the ridgeline and record their aging. "That's a camera," one of the watched characters breathes as they stare up the cliffs. "They're recording us." In a film, time is experiential as well as objectified. Cinematic time intermittently flows and freezes. Indeed, there is a dizzying moment in which the children chase each other in a game of freeze tag. The camera dollies through the sand, moving alongside the subject, and then it stops, suddenly, to contemplate the cinematically mummified figure at a distance. In this scene, the audience exists both inside of the film's temporal flow and, for a brief moment at least, outside of it, observing the film's movements from afar. The conundrum is that one never stops aging; time always passes, even during these "frozen" moments. Shyamalan's spectator is therefore implicated in the lived temporality of his film. In a revelation that must be troubling, if only because the film concerns a rapidly aging population, to watch *Old* is to enter, in many cases unwittingly, into "an encompassing temporal situation" from which there can no escape but to reach its terminus (Carruthers 2016: 29).

Reliant on the foundational work of Bazin, Lee Carruthers insists that film spectatorship "shows us time, not as something we know in advance, or master retrospectively, but as an ambiguous event that is opened up in experience" (ibid: 20). Shyamalan's *Old* enacts this ambiguous event by implicating the spectator in the experience of cinematic time not as something to be analyzed from afar, but something to be lived, in "real time." Carruthers employs the term timeliness to describe the immersive experience of time in a given film: "Timeliness frames the effort to enter into the temporal event that the film generates – because enduring that event, from start to finish, is itself a meaningful issue" (34). In the closing moments of *Old*, Shyamalan's spectator watches as waves slowly wash away debris on the beach. Having solved the puzzle of the beach at last, the two survivors swim through a strange reef, successfully evading the gaze of the scientist upon the hill (played by Shyamalan himself). Shyamalan's character stands behind an exaggerated camera lens, befuddled; the gaze of the film, too, scans the horizon, no longer able to track the characters. The spectator is meant to presume, however momentarily, that the sibling survivors have perished at sea. What endures beyond the frame? Or, more to the point, is there a way of being in time that exists outside of cinematic time?

The final shot of the film suggests that important lessons can be gleaned from Shyamalan's unique timeliness: the camera gradually drifts away from a helicopter in which the survivors must now re-orient themselves to a different experience of time, to a cadence that has not been set by meddlesome directors. The closing shot insists that the spectator look down upon the ocean, just as Shyamalan's enlightened characters stare outward into the blue beyond at the twilight of their lives, and she might (or so the logic of the film posits) start to appreciate a less plotted sense of being in time. As a character comments, "I want to be here... right now." For Shyamalan, cinema can heighten a spectator's fear of aging, but it can also alleviate this sense of existential dread by empowering the spectator to overcome their obsessions with past and future and embrace a deeper present. In other words, Shyamalan's spectator too could gaze gratefully upon the ebbs and flows of cinematic time instead of striving to solve the (impossible) "problem" of old age – a "problem" posited in mortal as well as aesthetic terms.

Author Bio

Michael J. Blouin is a Professor of English and Humanities at Milligan University. He is the author of the book *Japan and the Cosmopolitan Gothic: Specters of Modernity*. His recent works include *Democracy and the American Gothic* (forthcoming) as well as *Stephen King and American Politics*. He lives in East Tennessee with his partner and two daughter.

Works Cited

Bazin, Andre (2004): "The Ontology of the Photographic Image." In Leo Braudy and Marshall Cohen (eds.), *Film Theory and Criticism: Sixth Edition*, Oxford, UK: Oxford University Press, pp. 166–170.

Brooks, Peter (1984): *Reading for the Plot: Design and Intention in Narrative*, New York: Knopf.

Carruthers, Lee (2016): *Doing Time: Temporality, Hermeneutics, and Contemporary Cinema*, Albany, NY: SUNY Press.

Collier, Patrick C. (2008): "'Our Silly Lies': Ideological Fictions in M. Night Shyamalan's 'The Village.'" In: *Journal of Narrative Theory*, vol. 38, no. 2, pp. 269–92.

Hoy, David Couzens (2012): *The Time of Our Lives: A Critical History of Temporality*, Cambridge, MA: MIT Press.

Kermode, Frank (2000): *The Sense of an Ending: Studies in the Theory of Fiction*, Oxford, UK: Oxford University Press.

Lady in the Water. Directed by M. Night Shyamalan, Performances by Paul Giamatti and Bryce Dallas Howard, Warner Bros., 2006.

Lim, Bliss Cua (2009): *Translating Time: Cinema, The Fantastic, and Temporal Critique*, Durham, NC: Duke University Press.

Old. Directed by M. Night Shyamalan, Performances by Gael Garcia Bernal and Vicky Krieps, Universal Pictures, 2021.

Rosen, Philip (2001): *Change Mummified: Cinema, Historicity, Theory*, Minneapolis, MN: University of Minnesota Press.

The Village. Directed by M. Night Shyamalan, Performances by William Hurt and Sigourney Weaver, Touchstone Pictures, 2004.

The Visit. Directed by M. Night Shyamalan, Performances by Olivia DeJonge, Ed Oxenbould, Blumhouse, 2015.

Wollen, Peter (2004): "The Auteur Theory." In Leo Braudy and Marshall Cohen (eds.), *Film Theory and Criticism: Sixth Edition*, Oxford, UK: Oxford University Press, pp. 565–581.

A Horrifying Reversal
The Dislocating Impact of Age Consciousness in "The Curious Case of Benjamin Button"

Michael S. D. Hooper[1]

Introduction

The rediscovery, and subsequent release of George Romero's public-service film *The Amusement Park* offers a timely reminder of ageism's longevity and of the way that aging in American culture is often paired with Gothic horror. Created in 1973 at the behest of the Lutheran Service Society of Western Pennsylvania – and then rejected because it was too radical – *The Amusement Park* depicts a widespread assault on older Americans by the younger generations – anything from fleecing them out of their once cherished possessions to coercing them into institutions that stigmatize and aggravate their physical incapacities. A metaphor for an uncaring and increasingly bewildering modern America, the amusement park renders its older visitors disoriented and lost, a process that centers on the film's narrator and only professional actor, Lincoln Maazel. This septuagenarian, responsible for communicating the film's central message about age discrimination, is forced to encounter his double – a battered, bloodied, disheveled version of himself that registers the film's many setbacks for its older citizens. Dressed in white, he is both spectral and a prominent victim, for, as Richard Brody notes, the film, and especially its setting, carries the "crucial implication

---

[1] Independent Scholar.

that the social isolation of old age endures even in very public spaces" (2021). This estrangement is underscored by a series of "carnivalesque disturbances" (ibid.), Romero (already having directed *Night of the Living Dead* by this point) realizing that "the essence of horror isn't grotesquerie or gore but the sense of a world in dysfunction" (ibid.). Uncomfortable close-ups and jarring sound effects force the viewer to identify with the film's victims, to comprehend the multifarious ways in which an aged body is abused and made to feel superfluous.

This idea of dysfunction is also central to a short story published some 50 years before *The Amusement Park* and also about age or more precisely the, for many, terrifyingly uncontrollable process of aging. F. Scott Fitzgerald's "The Curious Case of Benjamin Button" (1922), by no means original in its employment of reverse chronology, postulates the frightening coincidence of extreme old age and childhood, playing on fears of congenital abnormality and the horror trope of the monstrous birth; and, in its preoccupation with time and the life course, reflects early 20th-century anxieties about both regulation and age consciousness.[2] As in *The Amusement Park*, the aged body, is viewed as contemptible, but here it is more unmistakably a freak, a *puer senex*, that disgusts and is rejected, its surprising proximity to childhood offering only a reminder of perceived similarities between senility and early infancy.

Often seen as whimsical and labeled by its author as one of his "fantasies" (Fitzgerald 2002: 6), "The Curious Case of Benjamin Button" has an underlying gravity that reflects not the euphoria and optimism of the post-World War I years but, instead, a discomfort with the (at the time) recent recognition of life stages and a profound sadness at the loss of a generation of fighting men. And it achieves this in part through a horror pastiche, by embodying age in a way which renders it simultaneously disgusting and absurd because, after all, "Gothic formulas readily produce laughter as abundantly as emotions of terror or horror" (Botting 2014: 174). A diluted form of the "shudder art" (1983: 41) that James B.

---

2 On the subject of originality, Fitzgerald himself acknowledged that Samuel Butler had already created "an almost identical plot" (Fitzgerald 2002: 7) in his *Notebooks* (1912).

Twitchell sees as an intermittent barometer of society's fears and their resolution, "The Curious Case of Benjamin Button" is, I will argue, not only unlike the stories of Fitzgerald's more usual social-realist mode, but also noticeably different from the handful of Gothic tales that feature ghosts or supernatural presences.

The acclaimed 2008 film adaptation of the short story, directed by David Fincher and with a screenplay written by Eric Roth, is also relevant here. Both departing from and extending the original in so many ways, this better-known version of the story nonetheless picks up on the connection between time/age and horror in frame stories that depict the unconscionable loss of life in World War I, and the ecological terror posed by Hurricane Katrina in 2005. In doing so, it highlights the way in which Fitzgerald's story was not simply a piece of escapism, an eccentric speculation but, beneath the sometimes-flippant tone of its narrator, a story borne of uncertainty and fear.

Age Consciousness

The transition to a life of increasing age consciousness at the end of the 19th century and the beginning of the 20th has been well documented, not least by the social historian Howard Chudacoff in his book *How Old Are You? Age Consciousness in American Culture* (1989). In a range of areas and ways, Chudacoff explains, Americans became more aware of distinct phases of life and, consequently, of peer groups, "institutionalized transitions [...] replacing rites of passage and regularizing the process of role assumption" (1989: 27). An improvement in survival rates facilitated this, but the impact of the Industrial Revolution was also considerable. The new machine age brought with it a demand for greater productivity and a concomitant acceptance that those in what were considered their advanced years could contribute little and had to be removed from the workforce. The establishment of retirement, part of a newly separate period of senescence, was complemented at the other end of the age spectrum by the creation of the branch of pediatric medicine, the formal recognition of adolescence and, following the extension of educational provision to the young, greater differentiation between school year groups, culminating in the creation of the junior high school. Beyond school, societies and organizations like the YMCA cemented the idea that the young had their own spheres of interest that required their own time and space; they could no longer be lumped together with adults in an attempt to accelerate their development and propel them into the world of work. Time, too, took on a whole new meaning. The increased regulation of working hours inevitably affected leisure time, more people relying on clocks and watches to set their routines than on daylight hours. And the passing of extended periods of time was marked by the more frequent observance and celebration of birthdays and other anniversaries.

Fundamental shifts in concepts of age and time were, then, altering the lives of individuals and the American population as a whole. While these changes lent greater clarity to the life cycle, a reassuring sense of shared experiences between peers for some, there was also the more unavoidable realization that a life was being measured in terms of usefulness and that its final phase could, with little state aid for the elderly, be precarious. Additionally, the way in which the phase of senescence had been determined by medical practitioners – by emphasizing the inevitability of ever worsening physical infirmities and the probability of mental decline – meant that the respect older Americans had previously commanded was being challenged, making way, certainly by the post-World War 1 years, for the veneration of youth. As Kirk Curnutt explains, "the 1920s associated maturation with decline and fretted over what experiences could render one 'old'" (2007: 30). F. Scott Fitzgerald was at the center of this – fretting, yes, but also riding high on the wave of his youthful celebrity and creating characters for whom the pursuit of hedonism was a natural affirmation of their immature outlooks. For, "age was his chief index of integrity" (ibid: 29) and a constant reference point in Fitzgerald's frequently overlapping life and fiction.

Outside of "Benjamin Button," the Fitzgerald story most concerned with age consciousness and the policing of age-appropriate behavior is arguably "At Your Age". Published in 1929, this often overlooked tale of a middle-aged man, Tom Squires, and his on-off relationship with a much younger woman, Annie Lorry, perfectly captures the conflict between societal prejudices to age difference and the individual's fluctuating belief in both his own vitality and his ability to offer experience and protection as a compensation for lost youth. The very title of the story implies that there is something undignified in an older man's pursuit of youthful relationships, and yet Tom seems unable to help himself as his first encounter with a blonde sales assistant in a drugstore, through to his reunion with Annie after a brief separation, shows. Moreover, following the aforementioned emphasis on productivity, the protagonist views his life in phases and with cut-off points: "'In ten years I'll be sixty, and then no youth, no beauty for me ever any more'" (Fitzgerald 1989: 486). Like a working life, his romantic career will cease at a precise point, leaving him dead to anything he values. As Tom sets about exploiting this last lease of romantic life to the full, "relishing the very terminology of young romance" (ibid: 490), Fitzgerald uses the seasons to show not a late blooming but a desperate clinging to a prolonged winter. It is already summer when Annie's inevitable drift towards more youthful companions occurs and Tom has his epiphany: "Tom realized with a shock that he and her mother were people of the same age looking at a person of another." (ibid: 493) The pursuit of youth has blinded him to the obvious, and the age consciousness of the time has left him looking foolish. Tom's only consolation is now nostalgia: returning to his childhood haunts, as he does at the end of the story, and locking in the memory of his three months with Annie Lorry – proof that he has been "used up a little" (ibid: 494) before death.

"At Your Age" is not a Gothic story but it satirizes the way that society views significant age difference in romantic/sexual relationships as monstrous, and its very precise classifications indicate just how far age awareness had permeated the population. Tom Squires is only fifty, but, with "his cheeks a little leathery and veined" (ibid: 487), he cuts a lonely figure, despite the considerable wealth he has accrued since the war and his earlier reputation as a highly eligible socialite. And it is this isolation that Fitzgerald exposes so poignantly in the brief final section of "At Your Age," conceding, as he does, the idea that there is a "penalty for age's unforgivable sin – refusing to die" (ibid: 494).

Echoes of the Gothic

Fitzgerald's Gothicism mainly stems from his use of ghosts, supernatural presences, and unnerving settings in the later sections of his narratives. "The Ice Palace" (1920) and "A Short Trip Home" (1927), for example, explore familiar themes of romance and social class before abruptly shifting into scenes of terror, bewilderment, and spectral possession. "One Trip Abroad" (1930), a story of gradual dissipation and boredom away from America, takes an eerie turn in its final paragraphs as its central characters, Nicole and Nelson Kelly, realize that the shadowy couple they have intermittently seen throughout the story are their doppelgängers, confirming both their togetherness and their social isolation. The Gothic impulse is restrained in all of these stories and yet it can make the writing seem forced, as if a final effect or scene is trying to surprise or shock the reader almost at the expense of narrative coherence. Preferring the wider, catch-all term of "fantasy," many of Fitzgerald's critics have, according to Derek Lee, "ignored these works or regarded them as side experiments in didacticism, allegory, and nonsense, rather than as a serious aesthetic strategy" (2018: 126). Lee himself tries to resurrect Fitzgerald's "latent supernaturalism" (ibid.) in the belief that it is entirely consistent with the influence of various forms of Romanticism on the writer and with the purpose of revealing "the social excesses of modernity" (ibid.: 133). If Fitzgerald's Gothic stories are clichéd or over the top, it is, he maintains, because the form demands them to be, the logical conclusion of this being the denouement of "One Trip Abroad" in which "the corruption of a Romantic ideal into Gothic blight is so excessive and lurid that only a supernatural epiphany can rectify what standard didactic storytelling cannot" (ibid.).

Though he considers Gothic elements in the longer fiction – *This Side of Paradise* (1920) and *Tender is the Night* (1934) – Lee overlooks "Benjamin Button," only noting Kim Sasser's magic-realist reading of this story which brings together irony and horror. Sasser herself acknowledges that "Benjamin Button" has "a peculiarly ambiguous relationship with literary classification" (2010: 181), hence her willingness to find connections between the various genres of American fable, fairy tale, fantasy, and satire. Magic realism, Sasser argues, provides a single framework for the interpretation of a story that carries no authorial comment on its supernatural events. Ultimately, though, Fitzgerald's social critique lies behind the story's playfulness, his target being, according to Sasser, the upper class and its obsession with reputation. While we might expect characters, including his parents, to be "absolutely dismayed at Benjamin's ontology" (Sasser 2010: 196), they are, instead, worried about how his inexplicable abnormality could derail their success and blemish their status within the upper echelons of Baltimore society in which the story is set. This highly plausible reading of the text means that the reverse chronology of Benjamin's life is an implicit questioning of Neoliberalist progress: social complacency might be concealing the fact that advancement is, in truth, a form of regression. Yet the parity Sasser finds between technique and purpose does not explain the value of time and age per se, only the ways they symbolize the failures of the most socially privileged.

Fitzgerald's own account of the origins of "Benjamin Button" would seem to support both an attack on social pretension and a questioning of the different life stages. In *Tales of the Jazz Age*, he admitted that the story "was inspired by a remark of Mark Twain's to the effect that it was a pity that the best part of life came at the beginning and the worst part at the end" (Fitzgerald 2002: 7). A humorist known for his witty remarks and opposition to discrimination and inequality, Twain seems to be highlighting a curious given and a manmade injustice. Even from his 19th-century perspective, he can surely see beyond biological decline to society's stigmatizing of those no longer automatically respected for their experience and acquired wisdom.

Fitzgerald converts this prejudice into horror, albeit with a light touch that suggests perversity and freakishness rather than genuine supernatural eeriness. The uncanny spectrality of the Gothic stories mentioned above is supplanted by a cringeworthy corporeality in "Benjamin Button," by – following Xavier Aldana Reyes's recent redefinition of the term – a form of body horror. Expanding its usual designation of extreme mutilation in splatter movies and splatterpunk, Aldana Reyes proposes five distinct, but potentially overlapping, forms of body horror, the grotesque being one of these and the most pertinent here. This variation of the subgenre is, according to the critic, "productively separated from other manifestations of body horror because its 'monstrous' bodies are intelligibly human, their 'otherness' a gross extension or exaggeration of the normative body" (2022: 112). As we will see, a character like Benjamin Button is abject rather than abhuman, his "gross extension" being the oscillating captivity of youth and age in respectively contrasting bodies, a violation of natural laws that is bizarre and puzzling rather than fantastic or supernatural.

Fitzgerald's story takes the simple but unexpected conceit of a life lived backwards, one which begins inauspiciously in 1860 and ends quietly in 1930, Benjamin Button having become a baby with little sense of the world around him. At each stage, this trajectory records how Benjamin is out of step with those who should be his peers. He is, for example, chased out of Yale by hordes of mocking students who view his attempted registration as an act of willful lunacy. Similarly, his army commission is greeted with incredulity at every turn, from the military outfitter to the colonel who sends him home. Usually, Benjamin is a hapless victim, visibly too old or too young for a situation, but in his married life we see how age first works to his advantage and then how he responds to its negative signs, having been infected by society's assumptions and prejudices with regard to age discrepancies. Benjamin marries Hildegarde Moncrief who is "beautiful as sin" (Fitzgerald 2002: 182) and the daughter of General Moncrief. While Annie Lorry seems merely to accept the temporary affections of Tom Squires in "At Your Age," Hildegarde offers a very full justification of her attraction to mature, fifty-year-old men: "'You're just the romantic age,' she continued – 'fifty. Twenty-five is too worldly-wise; thirty is apt to be pale from overwork; forty is the age of long stories that take a whole cigar to tell; sixty is – oh, sixty is too near seventy; but fifty is the mellow age. I love fifty.'" (ibid: 183) The irony that Benjamin is only twenty at this point is not lost on either him or the reader. Nevertheless, Hildegarde's classification flies in the face of convention as the extraordinary public and media outcry at their engagement proves. And it is not reciprocated by Benjamin himself. Predictably, he loses interest is his wife, finding her physically and behaviorally dull and his home a stifling prison from which he must escape. Once Benjamin's champion, Hildegarde drifts out of the story and has no part in his second childhood.

Monstrous Beginnings

Fitzgerald's narrator employs the opening section of his story to suggest the monstrously unnatural and to satirize the quintessential Gothic birth. The split between home and a more public space, one which the story consistently makes, underscores the idea that there is a proper, natural place for childbirth (although this may change over time) and that the Buttons have injudiciously ignored this. Moreover, home, where the birth should have occurred, is then, following the instructions of the nurse, to be a site of concealment and privacy in contradistinction to the openness and visibility of the medical establishment. Benjamin is a monstrous mistake that needs to be hidden away but not destroyed: "'This is your child, and you'll have to make the best of it'" (ibid: 172–3), the nurse comments somewhat accusingly. Yet Benjamin has, of course, to be transported home and this provokes further horror, this time in the mind of his father: "A grotesque picture formed itself with dreadful clarity before the eyes of the tortured man – a picture of himself walking through the crowded streets of the city with this appalling apparition stalking by his side." (ibid: 173) Following the lead of the physician and nurse, Roger Button internalizes a sense of both shame and outrage; his own son, for whom he has harbored lofty aspirations like a Yale education, is an aged doppelgänger, part of a Gothic nightmare built on the inseparability of public scorn and abnormality ("appalling," "stalking").

A cluster of references to time – "As long ago as 1860," "fifty years ahead of style," "one day in the summer of 1860," "this anachronism" (ibid: 169) – knits together chronology and the unusual, both distancing us from the events (supposedly occurring 60 years before the story is written) and drawing us into a world where time is a new imperative. The narrator, rooted in the chronopolitics of 1922, is, understandably in a reverse fictional biography, preoccupied with sequencing and correlating

Benjamin's actual age with his physical one. This continues throughout the story's eleven sections, but is especially noticeable at the beginning where time, abnormality, and reputation/status coalesce to create overwhelming feelings of disgust and anger. As a first-time father, Roger Button is understandably nervous.[3] His apprehension is heightened, however, by the family physician, Dr Keene, who is first glimpsed "rubbing his hands together with a washing movement" (ibid.). Physically and metaphorically abnegating his Hippocratic responsibility, the doctor, like the nurse Roger subsequently encounters, is moved to irritation and a feeling of being unfairly imposed upon. The tone is one of humor, created by "a satirical-comedic [narrative] voice" (Curnutt et al 2009: 5), exasperated comments, quizzical facial expressions, and even slapstick in the form of a basin slipping out of the nurse's hands and dropping down the stairs, yet the language also captures a sense of effrontery and horror. The doctor is, as befits the story's title, initially noted as having "a curious expression" and as "throwing a curious glance" (ibid: 170), as if his own demeanor has been upset by the unprecedented birth over which he has presided. This, though, soon gives way to "a perfect passion of irritation" (ibid: 170) and a feeling of indignation (the blustered "outrageous" is echoed by the nurse, ibid: 170 and 171).

Parodying the foundational Gothic birth, that of the creature in Mary Shelley's *Frankenstein* (1818), Fitzgerald emphasizes a nascent hostility to old age and an increasing anxiety about aging into irrelevance in the 1920s sensibility. Where Victor Frankenstein is crushed by "the accomplishment of my toils" (Shelley 1996: 34), an unsightly and apparently lifeless Adam that symbolizes both the scientist's misguided overreaching, the "ardour that far exceeded moderation" (ibid.), and genuine 19th-century fears about infant mortality and congenitally cursed children, Roger Button, enjoying the highest of social and financial privileges, is made to feel that a much longed for parenthood is a cruel joke. Personal shame engenders the instinct to reject, even to walk away. Incredibly, Frankenstein interprets a detaining hand as an act of aggression and

---

3   The birth of the Fitzgeralds' first and only child, Frances Scott (Scottie), on October 26, 1921, is often overlooked in relation to this story.

takes "refuge in the court-yard belonging to the house which I inhabited" (ibid: 35) – noticeably not a bona fide home, either, and a symbol of the scientist's repudiation of domesticity. Mary Shelley leaves us in little doubt that he is attempting to extricate himself from a problem – "the demoniacal corpse to which I had so miserably given life" (ibid.) – of his own creation. Similarly, Roger Button, solely influenced by the physician's disbelief and anger, is reluctant to go to the hospital and only mounts its steps with "the greatest difficulty" (Fitzgerald 2002: 170–1).

Both writers use attempts at speech as a means of reinforcing strangeness and to insist on their thematic concerns. Frankenstein's creature, born without the power of recognizable language, nevertheless opens his jaws and mutters "some inarticulate sounds" (Shelley 1996: 35) accompanied by a grin that "wrinkled his cheeks" (ibid.). With less conviction, we are told that "he might have spoken, but I did not hear" (ibid.). Fear and the father's determination to reject combine to nullify communication, no matter how unintelligible. Later, of course, in his own narrative, we learn how articulate the Noble Savage has become as he locates and expounds, with admirable honesty and sensitivity, on the trauma of being spurned by a parent. Here, though, the uncertainty of communication seems more attributable to Frankenstein's unwillingness to allow the creature a voice which might assert his humanity; and to a conviction that this travesty of a creation is innately malevolent as evidenced by the grin that noticeably wrinkles an already unsightly appearance. The seeds of revenge and destruction, important themes in *Frankenstein*, are already sown in these quick, judgemental encounters.

In Fitzgerald's story, Benjamin disarms – and makes a comic situation still more absurd – by speaking assuredly of the indignities he has encountered already: the interminable howling of babies and the inadequate blanket in which he has been swaddled. Though his voice is "cracked and ancient" (Fitzgerald 2002: 172), Benjamin is able to repeatedly express the stereotypical impatience of an older person in an unfamiliar milieu. Humorously unexpected and lucid, his objections allude to an increasing separation according to age – in particular, perhaps, the growing tendency to place older citizens in poorhouses or the relatively few nursing homes that existed when Fitzgerald wrote the story. Further, Benjamin's unwelcome presence in the hospital indicates an increasing discomfort with age in a period, the 1920s, when youth was garnering so much appeal; and his desire to extract himself and have his comforts and frailties at least recognized points to the more visible age stratification affecting American lives from approximately 1850 onwards.

The speech, or attempted speech, of a newborn is, by definition, unnerving, further reminding the reader of the simultaneity of age and extreme youth, and of the conspicuous absence of innocence. Labeled an "imposter" (ibid.) by his father, Benjamin is no changeling, the presence of which can be attributed to supernatural factors; rather, he is, as the nurse confirms, Mr Button's burden, and, more figuratively, the focus of anxieties about time's new importance and how it was profoundly continuing to redraw intergenerational relationships in the early part of the 20th century.

Losing a Generation

Mark Twain's fanciful invitation to rearrange the life cycle so that we can better enjoy our advanced years takes on new meaning in the aftermath of World War I. The immediate relief at the cessation of hostilities was qualified by dislocation and uncertainty: the realization that the war signified an irrevocable break with the past. Unofficially, Fitzgerald became part of the Lost Generation, one of a group of writers, that included Ernest Hemingway and Gertrude Stein, whose work reflected the vacuum and indirection at the heart of Western culture. Unable to imagine the full carnage of war, Fitzgerald "concentrates on the bitter peace" (Meredith 2004: 165), especially, as James H. Meredith notes, in another story from *Tales of the Jazz Age*, "May Day" (1920), nominally about "prosperity impending" (Fitzgerald 2002: 61) but actually concerned with the aggression that war has "unleashed at home" (Meredith 2004: 176).

Published just four years after the end of the Great War, "The Curious Case of Benjamin Button" mentions three conflicts – the Civil War, the Spanish-American War, and World War I – but at no point does the story explicitly gauge the toll these take on American life. The Civil War, ostensibly the reason for transporting us back to 1860, creates a minor subtext of slavery and difference. The war preoccupies Baltimore society at a time when awkward questions might be asked about the Buttons' progeny that would affect their standing. It also clarifies Roger Button's glib racism as, speculating on a journey of shame past the slave market, he expresses the wish of "a dark instant" (Fitzgerald 2002: 173) that his son was black. Benjamin's bravery and rapid promotion during the Spanish-American War of 1898 lead to his World War 1 call-up and a prized commission as brigadier-general. At this point, though, Benjamin's younger physical age makes his authority preposterous and he is literally stripped of his uniform.

The character's motivation for, and non-participation in, the Great War parallels Fitzgerald's own experience. Just as Benjamin views combat as a means of escaping his suffocating home life (especially his marriage), so Fitzgerald willingly enlisted to avoid further failure at Princeton. The novelist was about to depart for France when the war ended, denying him the heroism he also sought. It seems likely, though, that, following his experiences at various training camps, Fitzgerald would have proved a less than competent officer. Jeffrey Meyers, one of his biographers, talks of a military life characterized by "escapades and disasters" (2000: 39), and, more damningly, spells out the writer's ignorance: "Fitzgerald, who was extremely self-absorbed, had no serious interest in or understanding of the greatest historical event of his lifetime: World War 1." (2000: 34) Meyers refers, by way of support, to the strikingly brief section labeled "Historical" in the second chapter of the loosely autobiographical *This Side of Paradise* where the narrator's "studied indifference" (2000: 34) to what he dismisses as "an amusing melodrama" (Fitzgerald 1995: 58) is all too apparent.

Though "Benjamin Button" glosses World War I, it does so because its protagonist's physical and chronological age are both outside of the parameters set for active service and not because the war is either too irrelevant or too horrific to contemplate. Yet the conjunction of war and age is a moot one: a youthful generation was decimated by the bloodiest and most protracted of conflicts. A life lived in reverse, one that has the good fortune to elude the horrific (predominantly European) sacrifice, approaches and harnesses youth in the face of historical inevitability and, in the process, once again indirectly highlights the salience of time and age differentiation. Behind Fitzgerald's fantastical premise is a desire to privilege youth but also to reverse history itself.

This is something that assumes a more romantic dimension four years later in *The Great Gatsby* where the deluded hero believes not only that time can be reversed – to a point preceding Daisy's marriage to Tom Buchanan – but also that he can create a facsimile of the past. Indeed, even in a state of heightened anxiety, Gatsby symbolically controls time, catching Nick Carraway's mantelpiece clock during his awkward first reunion with Daisy. Of more direct relevance here, though, is David Fincher's film adaptation of "Benjamin Button" which completely alters the timeframe of Fitzgerald's story. The Armistice that signaled the end of Fitzgerald's own military pretensions becomes the commencement of Benjamin's initially inauspicious life, and celebratory fireworks light up the night sky as Mr Button first runs to the birth of his child (in the family home, not a hospital) and then seeks a means of disposing of him. The end of World War I is the distraction the Civil War provides in Fitzgerald's story, except here almost no one at this point knows of Benjamin's existence and the viewer has not even been privileged with a glimpse of the baby hidden by its blanket. It is not an ironic counterpoint to disappointment and death (Mrs Button dies in childbirth) because of the film's other frame story: the building of a new train station, complete with a new clock, in New Orleans (where this version of the story is set) also in 1918.[4] Mr Gateau, blind but the greatest horologist in the South and still grieving the death of his son in the war, creates a timepiece that moves backwards to resurrect a generation of young men: "I made it that way … so that perhaps the boys that we lost in the war might stand and come home again …" (Roth 2008: 40). Granting his wish, this story subsequently includes footage of ammunition leaving soldiers' bodies and returning to weapons – proof that art can salvage life and manipulate

---

4   This story is narrated by Daisy, Benjamin's former lover, before Caroline, their daughter, reads Benjamin's journal and before we, in turn, hear his voiceover.

time in the way that Twain theorized and Fitzgerald realized in his short story. The practicality of timekeeping in the modern age, as necessary at a train terminus as anywhere else, is juxtaposed with a fantasy that encapsulates one man's grief and a nation's loss. The element of horror that the original short story circumvented by having Benjamin miss the war is manifest here and compounded by the reaction of the gathered crowd. Instead of being moved by Mr Gateau's story, the people do not know how to react, caught as they are between respect for the dead and outrage that the new clock does not function properly. In this way, then, Roth and Fincher are able to tease out of Fitzgerald's story the writer's critique of the hegemonic centrality of time and his unstated lament for a lost generation of men for whom youth was barely experienced.

Born in 1918 in Fincher's film, Benjamin Button simultaneously connotes, in his aged incarnation, the unattainable life beyond youth for so many World War I soldiers and the bewilderment of the postwar years – a pervasive disenchantment that Fitzgerald felt more acutely than the horrors of the war itself and which, of course, was most powerfully captured by T. S. Eliot's *The Waste Land*, published in the same year as the original short story. Fincher's film, though, neither begins with Benjamin's birth nor concludes with his death. Instead, advancing events to just before the film's creation, we follow the dying moments of Benjamin's former lover, Daisy, as she lies in a New Orleans hospital bed while Hurricane Katrina rages outside. Daisy's death is a formality but what is less certain is whether, as the custodian of Benjamin's story, she will survive its retelling.

Katrina echoes the tempestuous, action-packed life at the center of the film. It further justifies the switch in setting from antebellum Baltimore in the story to post-World War 1 New Orleans in the film. Aside from the dramatic tension it brings, the hurricane's main function, however, seems to be to offer some larger correlative – ecological, climatic – to the extraordinary events of the protagonist's life. Apocalyptic, the freakish storm tears apart a world that has ignored climate change, a city that has become complacent about flood defences, and a nation dismissive of social/racial inequality. Though the characters in this frame story – Daisy, Caroline (Daisy and Benjamin's daughter), and

Dorothy Baker (a care worker) – have little sense of the hurricane's full impact, the way in which it will strengthen further beyond the running television news reports in the background, the privileged viewer knows the likelihood of evacuation, the huge death toll, and the magnitude of a salvage operation that will, in time, effectively see the city reborn. It is a horror narrative that complements the unpalatability of Benjamin's birth and his initial warehousing in a home for the elderly; it is also a lugubrious counterpoint to the tender but doomed love story that emerges as the central focus of the film – a very different relationship to the faltering marriage of Benjamin and Hildegarde in the original story.

In another respect, too, the environmental disaster is a tenuous link to Benjamin's life or, rather, the end of it. Both story and film move swiftly through the final years, arriving at an uncomfortable predicament pairing youth and memory loss. In the story this is not explicitly dementia, more the welcome departure of "troublesome memories" (Fitzgerald 2002: 194) and then the lyrical fading of "unsubstantial dreams from his mind as though they had never been" (ibid: 195). In the film, though, this fortuitous release is made more painful by Daisy's visits to a young Benjamin clearly living with the early stages of dementia. The viewer witnesses his destitution (he has been found living in a condemned building), incapacity, and seeping memories via another person, namely the love of Benjamin's life who, in a neat twist, has temporarily become the mother he never had. In the story, by contrast, Nana, a nursemaid, is now "the center of his tiny world" (ibid: 194), but she has not been mentioned before and the narrator continues to focus on Benjamin rather than give us access to her thoughts. Crucially, the film suggests that, old or young, dementia may be an inevitable final stage, ultimately an aphasia that connects youth and age.[5] The concurrent hurricane underscores the popular fear that aging and the neurological diseases that might be associated with it have become so visible in the 21st century that they warrant alarmist Gothic language and meteorological metaphors – silver tsunami, silent killer, Alzheimer's epidemic, for example.

---

5   The screenplay makes this explicit when Benjamin is described as "like an eight year old, or an old man old with onset Alzheimer's" (Roth 2008: 203).

Conclusion: "What horrible mishap had occurred?"

On a personal level, the polarization of youth and old age left F. Scott Fitzgerald in a double bind. The "enculturated pursuit of youth" (Curnutt 2002: 30) afforded a tremendous sense of well-being alongside commercial opportunities: the chance to spin further a youthful credo to like-minded consumers.[6] Equally, its brevity – youth appeared to be more compressed than ever – was destabilizing amidst a lingering sense that, for all their vital presence in the music, fashion, and social mores of the time, the young still had to defer to their *betters*. In the same year that "Benjamin Button" was published, 1922, Fitzgerald penned an article for *American Magazine* in which he confessed to an age-induced vulnerability or over sensitivity. "What I Think and Feel at 25" is written with a tongue-in-cheek tone but, nonetheless, it registers both pessimism and resentment that seniors run the world and do so with the "ponderous but shallow convictions" (Fitzgerald 2005: 25) of their heightened wisdom and experience.

Neither pure whimsy nor a fictional representation of Fitzgerald's views, "The Curious Case of Benjamin Button" is an amusement park of sorts, a hall of distorting mirrors through which its protagonist is ridiculed and rejected for his asynchronous existence, for his inability to integrate consistently and meaningfully into the spheres of public and private life. Perplexed in the extreme – "What horrible mishap had occurred?", "Where in God's name did you come from?" (ibid: 170 and 172) – Benjamin's father even imputes that supernatural forces must have been at play that would utterly justify the abdication of parenthood, although this, as we have noted, is somewhat misjudged. Given no diagnostic explanation for Benjamin's strange condition, we nonetheless recognize that the entrapment of extreme youth within extreme age is not so much

---

6 Fitzgerald's understanding of his market is evident in a letter of May 11, 1922 to his editor, Maxwell Perkins. Of *Tales of the Jazz Age*, he confidently asserts: "It will be bought by *my own personal public* [original emphasis] – that is, by the countless flappers and college kids who think I am a sort of oracle (Fitzgerald 1964: 158).

a depiction of the "outright fantastic" as a means of contemplating that which might more prosaically "threaten to exceed and transform the apparently inviolable cohesion of our physical state" (Aldana Reyes 2022: 112 and 107).

While it is true, as Scott Ortolano contends, that, despite aspersions and handicaps, Benjamin finds a way to get on, to become "a kind of proto-businessman... an embodiment of the efficient business ideology that was driving the economic production of the 1920s" (2012: 133), this means of surmounting alterity is necessarily evanescent, a passing consolation in the inexorable passage of time towards youth and extinction. On attaining extreme infancy, Benjamin enjoys a tranquility of not remembering, the words "no," "not," and "nothing" (Fitzgerald 2002: 195) creating a rhythm, a lullaby of calming absence. His enterprise and his wartime bravery fall away as easily as if they had never been, making his biography a fable, a passage of years without enduring legacy. His end is a harmonious one sharply at odds with the panic and anger that accompanied his birth, but his physical youth has, finally, been no more rewarding than that of his shocking maturity. As Rachael McLennan notes, the story (unlike its film treatment) "withholds happy resolutions and is unsparing in its treatment of Benjamin" (2014: 642).

The protagonist is, as the full title of the story and film would suggest, a curiosity: a medical/psychological conundrum or a mystery to be solved. For all the personal involvement its biography-cum-case study seems to invite, however, "Benjamin Button" dramatizes more allegorically the way in which time, the aging process, and age stratification have altered priorities, bringing about a realignment of households, schools, workplaces, and a rethinking of peer-group relationships – a cultural shift from a time, before 1850, when "age was more a biological phenomenon than a social attribute" (Chudacoff 1989: 9). Benjamin's dislocation registers the confusion of a period, in the 1920s, when thoughts of longevity and the promise of youth were compromised by the two great killers of the preceding years: the Great War and the Great Influenza Epidemic; it also acknowledges retrospectively the more accelerated journey to modernity, with all its exigencies, that transformed the second half of the 19th century.

David Fincher and Eric Roth move beyond this pivotal period in their film adaptation, stretching Benjamin Button's life across the still more rapidly evolving 20th century, a time in which largely uncontested and embedded age classifications have arguably created a greater chasm between old age and youth. Certainly, the film's casting and special effects, emphasizing a physical beauty in Benjamin that is nowhere present in the story, would seem to valorize the latter in much the same way that Fitzgerald and popular American culture did in the 1920s. Despite this, Eric Roth's screenplay also reaches for a moral message beneath its surface texture, trying to locate an overarching significance to the mishap that is Benjamin's life. Its regrettably anodyne and "folksy maxim" (Curnutt et al 2009: 7) – steered towards an audience largely unfamiliar with Fitzgerald's story – that life, however experienced, is about controlling time and destiny to ensure optimum fulfillment, only serves to underline the importance of the original Benjamin's true historicity, the horror of his victimhood in an age when life stages in America "were being defined with near-clinical precision" (Chudacoff 1989: 52).

Author Bio

Dr Michael S. D. Hooper is an independent scholar based in the UK. He is the author of *Sexual Politics in the Work of Tennessee Williams: Desire over Protest* (CUP, 2012) and of several articles that have appeared in the *Tennessee Williams Annual Review*, including "Painting His Nudes: Tennessee Williams's Homoerotic Art" (2019). Recent publications include the essays "A Spectral Future: Dementia and the Nonhuman in *Marjorie Prime*" in *Age and Ageing in Contemporary Speculative and Science Fiction*, edited by Sarah Falcus and Maricel Oró-Piqueras (Bloomsbury, 2023), and "Playing House: Spatiality, Home, and Privacy in the Theatre of Jennifer Haley" in *Revista de Estudios Norteamericanos*, edited by Noelia Hernando-Real and John S. Bak (University of Seville Press, 2023).

Works Cited

Aldana Reyes, Xavier (2022): "Body Horror." In: Stephen Shapiro and Mark Storey (eds.), *The Cambridge Companion to American Horror*, Cambridge: Cambridge University Press, pp. 107–119.
Botting, Fred (2014): *Gothic*, London: Routledge.
Brody, Richard (2021): "A Rediscovered Featurette from the Modern Master of Horror." *New Yorker*, June 11, 2021, https://www.newyorker.com/culture/the-front-row/a-rediscovered-featurette-from-the-modern-master-of-horror.
Chudacoff, Howard P. (1989): *How Old Are You? Age Consciousness in American Culture*, New Jersey: Princeton University Press.
Curnutt, Kirk (2002): "*F. Scott Fitzgerald, Age Consciousness, and the Rise of American Youth Culture.*" In: Ruth Prigozy (ed.), *The Cambridge Companion to F. Scott Fitzgerald*, Cambridge: Cambridge University Press, pp. 28–47.
Curnutt, Kirk (2007): *The Cambridge Introduction to F. Scott Fitzgerald*, Cambridge: Cambridge University Press.
Curnutt, Kirk, Prigozy, Ruth, Mangum, Bryant, West III, James L. W., Inge, M. Thomas, Beuka, Robert, Seidel, Kathryn Lee, Bilton, Alan (2009): "The Case Gets Curious: Debates on 'Benjamin Button', From Story to Screen." In: *The F. Scott Fitzgerald Review* 7, pp. 2–33.
Fitzgerald, F. Scott (1964): *The Letters of F. Scott Fitzgerald*, edited by Andrew Turnbull, London: Bodley Head.
Fitzgerald, F. Scott (1989): "At Your Age." In: Matthew J. Bruccoli (ed.), *The Short Stories of F. Scott Fitzgerald*, New York: Scribner, pp. 481–494.
Fitzgerald, F. Scott (1995): *This Side of Paradise*, edited by James L. W. West III, Cambridge: Cambridge University Press.
Fitzgerald, F. Scott (2002): "May Day." In: James L. W. West III (ed.), *Tales of the Jazz Age*, Cambridge: Cambridge University Press, pp. 61–114.
Fitzgerald, F. Scott (2002): "The Curious Case of Benjamin Button." In: James L. W. West III (ed.), *Tales of the Jazz Age*, Cambridge: Cambridge University Press, pp. 169–195.

Fitzgerald, F. Scott (2005): "What I Think and Feel at 25." In: James L. W. West III (ed.), *My Lost City: Personal Essays, 1920–1940*, Cambridge: Cambridge University Press, pp. 16–26.

Lee, Derek (2018): "Dark Romantic: F. Scott Fitzgerald and the Specters of Gothic Modernism." In: *Journal of Modern Literature* 41(4), pp. 125–142.

McLennan, Rachael (2014): "Aging, Adaptation, and the Curious Cases of Benjamin Button." In: *Literature/Film Quarterly* 42 (4), pp. 635–648.

Meredith, James H. (2004): "Fitzgerald and War." In: Kirk Curnutt (ed.), *A Historical Guide to F. Scott Fitzgerald*, New York: Oxford University Press, pp. 163–213.

Meyers, Jeffrey (2000 [1994]): *Scott Fitzgerald: A Biography*, New York: Cooper Square Press.

Ortolano, Scott (2012): "Changing Buttons: Mainstream Culture in Fitzgerald's 'The Curious Case of Benjamin Button' and the 2008 Film Adaptation." In: *The F. Scott. Fitzgerald Review* 10, pp. 130–152.

Romero, George (2021[1973]): *The Amusement Park*, https://www.shudder.com/movies/watch/the-amusement-park/286f545b09818c85.

Roth, Eric (2008): *The Curious Case of Benjamin Button Screenplay*. In: F. Scott Fitzgerald, Eric Roth and Robin Swicord, *The Curious Case of Benjamin Button: Story to Screenplay*, New York: Scribner, pp. 33–211.

Sasser, Kim (2010): "The Magical Realist Case for 'Benjamin Button'." In: *The F. Scott Fitzgerald Review* 8, pp. 181–207.

Shelley, Mary (1996): *Frankenstein: 1818 Text*, edited by J. Paul Hunter, New York: W. W. Norton.

Twitchell, James B. (1983): "*Frankenstein* and the Anatomy of Horror." In: *The Georgia Review* 37 (1), pp. 41–78.

There's No Cure
Failures of the Aged under Neoliberalism

Kaydee Corbin Anderson[1] and Ahoo Tabatabai[2]

> I just saw my middle daughter get married. She's talking about having kids now. I have two other kids talking about marriage. That's what I want. I want more time to spend with my family so that I can create memories for myself and for them. Ultimately, I'll lose those memories with this disease, but they won't. (Zarney 2021)

Those are the words of a 57-year-old man who has been living with symptoms of Alzheimer's for 6 years. The quote was featured in a magazine article about the 2021 United States Food and Drug Administration approval of a new drug that has proven to be surprisingly ineffective at treating the disease. Partaking in this 25% effective drug is framed in the piece as an act of selflessness on the part of a father for his children.

---

1 University of Missouri – Kansas City.
2 Columbia College.

The Old Monster

The representation of older adults in horror is unique in that the anxieties and fears reflected to the audience are sometimes the result of real biological processes blended with the paranormal, a substitute in most horror for the unknown. Old age has often been read as a symbol for the decaying body and death. The aged are often portrayed in extreme biological decline, the body presented as having betrayed itself. Culturally speaking, the aged are often depicted as incapable, forgetful, unproductive, and burdensome. In horror, the aged are permitted to act with intent, nefarious or otherwise. This dissonance created between a stereotypical older adult and the aged portrayal in horror is useful as a plot device in film because it makes it difficult initially to determine if the older adult should be considered a threat or a victim. We contend that old age in horror is more than the representations and assumptions of the aged body, however. We propose that old age is a carrier-vessel for various social fears . It is not possible to examine all these social fears in one setting. In this paper we examine how old age is coded as a marker of failure. Since our current cultural narrative of personhood privileges productivity and personal responsibility, old age, particularly accompanied by cognitive decline, represents a terrifying deviation.

We will use the films *Relic* and *The Taking of Deborah Logan* to illustrate how narratives of age and illness are rehashed, not necessarily by highlighting the proximity to death but by showcasing the failure to be productive. The 2014 American film *The Taking of Deborah Logan* is presented as a documentary/found footage film. Mia, a doctoral student, has been given funds to document the effect of Alzheimer's on Deborah Logan. Deborah is cared for by her daughter, Sarah. The family is in need of the stipend provided by Mia's grant, thus locking them into a mutually beneficial relationship. The 2020 Australian film *Relic* is centered around the character of Edna who goes missing at the beginning of the film. Her daughter, Kay, and granddaughter, Sam, come to take care of her. While Edna is not officially diagnosed in the film, it is clear that her condition has worsened. We chose these films because they serve as illustrative examples of the unquestioned values embedded in our social narratives.

Medicalization of Aging

Goldman emphasizes how important fictional narratives are in the cultural interpretations of disease. She argues that in the 1970s, the naming of Alzheimer's marked both the creation of a disease and a new identity. Sontag argues that diseases that have cures are just diseases, those that do not, like AIDS, about which she writes extensively, and Alzheimer's, remain carriers of everything we fear. "The most terrorizing illnesses are those perceived not just as lethal but as dehumanizing" (1978: 27), she argues. Aging-as-disease can be framed effectively using the rich history of the study of other diseases, as well as the study of disabilities as subjectivities, with particular attention to cognitive decline and disabilities. The connection between cognitive decline and aging itself has had an important history on which horror films, perhaps unwittingly, build.

Social Factors Influencing Normal Aging Versus a Symptom of a Disease

In 1838, senile dementia was distinguished from various other mental disorders by French psychiatrist Jean-Étienne-Dominique Esquirol (Aquilina and Hughes 2006: 144). At the time, the term "senile" was used in the medical field to differentiate between diseases contracted by the old versus those contracted by the young. For example, bronchitis became "senile bronchitis" when someone over the age of 65 was diagnosed (Ballenger 2006).

In 1907, neuropathologist Dr. Alois Alzheimer described a patient with symptoms including "delusions, severe memory loss, disorientation, language deficits, and behavioral disturbances" (Villain and Dubois 2019: 3). Three years later, Alzheimer's disease (AD) was distinguished by neuropsychiatrist and nosologist Dr. Emil Kraepelin as a "presenile dementia" (Holstein 1997; Villain and Dubois 2019). Categorizing the disease "presenile" was considered revolutionary as cases of dementia at the time were firmly diagnosed based on age of the patient. Someone with relative youth displaying the same symptoms would not otherwise be considered as a patient that could be diagnosed with senile dementia.

As only older people were diagnosed with dementia before the pathology of AD, the relationship between one's age and being diagnosed with the disease was assumed. As more AD cases were diagnosed, the question of cause became more salient. Two arguments from the discourse at the time emerged: (1) AD as part of "an intensification" of the "normal" aging process impacted by various social factors and (2) "senility" as a symptom of a disease (Ballenger 2006: 101; Holstein 1997).

The issue of whether AD or, more broadly, senile dementia was a distinct disease, or an "exaggeration of normal aging" was a topic explored by researchers since AD's discovery (Ballenger 2006: 101). The term "senile" was so often associated with older adults that some argued that aging was being pathologized. (Ballenger 2006). Instead, between the 1920s and the 1960s, the psychodynamic theory of dementia emphasized social and psychosocial factors as contributing factors to a diagnosis of dementia (Wilson 2014), and deemphasized the relationship between age and dementia. It was argued that "moral, hereditarian, anatomical, and physiological" conditions impacted vulnerability to the disease (Ballenger 2006: 82; Holstein 1997; Wilson 2014). Physicians blamed "morbid, vicious indulgences" if a patient had symptoms of dementia before old age citing that such indulgences "rob" the brain of time needed to repair, causing damage to the gray cortex and blood vessels in the brain (Holstein 1997). In another popular analogy at the time, the brain was compared to a machine with a limited amount of energy. As one moved through life, the energy source was expected to deplete at the same rate (Holstein 1997). Those who suffered from dementia, therefore, were thought to have spent the given energy at a rate that was too high (Ballinger 2006).

Historically, the duty of the individual to avoid disease was also a matter of morality. Ballenger describes a "moralization of health" during the antebellum period in which Protestants agreed that senility was a punishment for sins against God (2006: 17). From this perspective, even an aged brain was not necessarily a suitable brain for AD or dementia and, especially someone with relative youth, was considered not only individually negligent, but also morally compromised (Villain 2019).

A Symptom of a Disease

In the late 1960s, the broader concept of "senility" as it relates to dementia was once again redefined. The term "senility" was considered ageist in its use rather than helpful in the medical community (Ballenger 2006: 81; Butler 1975). A newfound interest in reframing dementia as a scientific rather than exclusively a social problem developed (Ballenger 2006). The center of this argument was, once again, the relationship between senility and the aging process. The psychodynamic model of dementia was being reexamined and the focus was being shifted from the process of aging itself to presenting mental deterioration as "a problem suitable for cutting-edge medical science" (Ballenger 2006: 82). Ballenger describes Alzheimer's disease as "one of the most frightening and devastating of diseases at both the personal and the societal level" (2006: 56). The new gerontological persuasion associated deterioration and disability in old age as the result of disease, not necessarily old age itself. The gerontological persuasion broadly defined senility as one of the fundamental problems of aging and also mandated gerontologists clearly define boundaries between normal aging and disease.

As discussed in further detail below, while the diagnosis may have problematic implications for someone with AD or dementia today, there are implicit benefits to diagnosis that cannot be ignored. In a society that privileges medical opinion, the AD construct as a disease insinuates the existence of a cure that must be sought out. It gives hope that the "disturbance" and "disruption" that accompanies the disease should be managed and is manageable (Behuniak 2011; Stafford 1991). Stafford argues that through pathologizing senility, the fear of losing control of the mind to nature (natural causes) is lessened (1991: 395). Further, the pathology allows the blame for inappropriate outbursts to shift to the disease itself rather than the individual. Presenting dementia as a "worse way to grow old", Chivers, notes that the diagnosis itself, when separated from normal aging, may provide a sense of relief in one who is growing old (2011: 60).

Loss of Self

The biomedical understanding of AD and dementia is only one aspect to the diagnosis itself. While the history of how it became pathologized is necessary to understand some of the stigma experienced by victims, it is essential to include cultural framing of the disease and the implications for those diagnosed with AD or dementia. There is much information in the discourse regarding a loss of self experienced in being diagnosed, and navigating the world with AD or dementia (Aquilina and Hughes 2006; Basting 2003; Buhuniak 2011; Herskovits 1995).

As the individual was once responsible for maintaining proper habits to avoid dementia, the fear and anxiety surrounding the diagnosis may also be influenced by individual responsibility for maintaining selfhood (Ballenger 2006). Alzheimer's disease can be described as a "disease double," a term used to describe the layers of stigma, rejection, fear, and group exclusion that those suffering with the "dreaded disease" must navigate, creating a double victimization (Scheper-Hughes and Lock 1986: 137 – 138). Herskovits (1995) notes that a central way to define the self leans heavily on cognitive function. That is one part of the self specifically under attack by AD.

It should be noted that not all research agrees with a total loss of selfhood. Sabat and Harré (1992) argue that while selfhood remains intact in the disease, the marginalization of people with dementia by others results in a loss of the social aspects of selfhood. Ballenger discusses accounts from family and caregivers for individuals with AD or dementia that describe an "essential humanity" and a "connection with their former lives" that victims still retain (2006: 154). The "social death," contributes to the loss of self (Ballenger 2006: 172).

Medicalization of aging has created an established standard for how to grow old. For example, the focus of retirement on leisure and being healthy enough to experience leisure correctly. With this new focus, new standards of being normal were also established. Failure to be a normal old person is a deviation. (Ballenger 2006: 9–10). The deviation from the expectation is frightening.

The "Monstering"

Within both medical discourse and popular culture, there exists a problematic language linking AD and "monsterization" or "dehumanization" of the victim (Aquilina and Hughes 2006: Buhuniak, 2011; Herskovits 1995). Examples can be found in the discourse describing AD for example as "the funeral without end," the loss of self," a "social death," victims as "living corpses" experiencing a "living death," the body having outlived the mind," and "the death before death" (Ballenger 2006: 22; Herskovits 1995: 148; Matthews 2006; Robertson 1991).

The effects of AD have been described as representing a loss of human qualities of a patient (Robertson 1991.) This fear can be found at various levels throughout US culture in media, literature, and film (Basting 2003; Chivers 2011). It is present in jokes about aging presenting forgetfulness as a "senior moment" or "early Alzheimer's." It is not surprising that this fear is also internalized by those who have the disease themselves (Basting 2003).

It is not just the description of those with AD as less than human, but the metaphorical comparison of people with AD to zombies that solidifies the fearful distinction between those with the disease and those without. It should be noted that the intent of discussing this discourse is not to disparage the zombie metaphor in reference to AD, but to consider the comparison and contemplate the impact of its use. Behuniak argues "the frightening... images of... zombies [through] popular and scholarly discourse have construct[ed those diagnosed with AD] as animated corpses and their disease as a terrifying threat to the social order" (2011: 72). The zombie is characterized as less than human, a creature with no brain power, no intellect, and no memory of a past human life. They have little to no ability to recognize relationships with others or build rapport. The very things that we fear in terms of AD impacting our memories, "the social death", "the loss of self", can be seen in the characterization of the zombie (Basting 2003). It becomes problematic in that not only do those suffering from AD go through this loss in some way, the "disease double" process they go through stigmatizes and others them further, constructing the victim of AD as a social zombie (Ballinger 2006).

Aquilina and Hughes discuss AD patients as being "reanimated" with anti-dementia drugs. They note that despite obvious signs that the person suffering from AD is alive they are often "treated as already dead and as walking corpses to be both pitied and feared" (2006: 143). Behuniak (2011) notes that when the brain has been "destroyed" by disease, the person "no longer exists as a person but only as a body to be managed" (Behuniak 2011: 74). Matthews notes that the victim of AD may have a body that is still seen as alive, but "the person 'inside' the body is experienced as dead, or as good as dead" (2006: 163).

Neoliberal Take on the Worthiness of Love: Care in a Capitalist Society

How we choose to make sense of a film, its form or narrative, depends on the particular socio-political environment in which we are situated. A neoliberal society is one where the dominant narratives rely on the presumably indisputable logic of the market. Economically, neoliberalism is associated with cuts to the social safety net through deregulation and privatization. As a cultural hegemony, neoliberalism idealizes independence, defined narrowly as economic productivity and personal responsibility (Bergeron 2009; Holst 2021; Reich 2014; Shuffelton 2013). Neoliberalism also demands predictable domesticity from interpersonal relationships (Halberstam 2011). Relationships are understood in terms of supply and demand. In any given society, as established by cultural and political systems, there is a "preferred self" (McGuigan 2014). Neoliberal capitalism has such a preferred self. The preferred self of neoliberalism is an independent rational actor. The self is in a constant state of improvement and production, both in the economic sphere but also in the "economies of care" (Luna 2018). Relationships are based on what the self can provide. What the self can provide can certainly be productive: material/financial. But it can also be reproductive: care work. Care work includes literal reproduction but also the work that is needed to maintain a population, including maintaining those who are not yet (children) or no longer (elderly, ill, disabled) productive or reproductive. Where the preferred self is the productive/reproductive rational actor, there is a reluctant space made for the less-than-preferred self. In fact, the presence of the "less-than-ideal" or what we call "failed self", akin to Goffman's spoiled identity (1963), serves as a means to highlight the deserving space given to the preferred way of being. Those who fail, the elderly, the ill, the disabled, must continue to exhibit their own preferred self. In fact boundaries for how to appropriately "do" illness, age, and disability abound. In a neoliberal society, "care is not tied to the state but to family members therefore people have to try to make themselves "lovable" (Jaffe 2021: 47). In this sense, those who fail to be preferred, must show their worthiness in other ways. They must be loving and lovable. But they must also embrace their diminished capacity, acknowledging loss, and grieving. That the way in which the aged or the disabled live is a different way of being is fundamentally disruptive and is challenged at every turn. Age is perpetually framed as decline and loss. Cognitive decline, which is not necessarily a part of aging, but is often framed as such is an example of "death-in-life" (Black 2014). Black's notion refers to the moment when one becomes aware of no longer experiencing the world as the other (in her case someone with a mental illness). In horror films, the aged become a symbol for this notion of death-in-life. Therefore, it is not death itself that is the source of terror. This we argue is true for two reasons. First, death can be beautiful and death at the end of a long, productive life, can be a source of celebration. Second, the majority of horror film viewers are not invited to identify with the old person. The old person, however sympathetic, is the other. Viewers are invited to identify with the caregivers. The caregivers experience death-in-life, by virtue of no longer sharing an understanding of the world with their mothers, despite sharing with them a physical one.

Those who predominantly do care work in the United States and around the world are women. It is not surprising that the two central relationships in each of the films are between older women and their daughters. Eldercare is often relegated to women, both in professional settings and in families (Robertson 2014). In the U.S. eldercare is done not only by women but specifically by women of color and immigrant women. Both these films also feature relationships between white women. In the United States, white women have for centuries represented the ideal victims, for whom the sympathy of the majority can be galvanized. The notion of white women as worthy victims is outside the scope of this paper but others have contributed significantly to this topic (See for example Stillman 2007).

In both films, the lack of productivity of the women, Edna and Deborah, is illustrated through 1) their inability to care for their bodies, as a stand-in for the decline of the mind, 2) inability to care for their homes and 3) inability to maintain relationships, i.e. live up to what is expected of them as women who are caregivers, and also inability to make themselves "lovable" enough to be cared for.

Inability to Care for Bodies and Minds

Each woman is shown to physically decline. The mental decline is the forefront of the story, but the physical decline becomes a way to visualize personhood-diminished. Deborah specifically is shown as traditionally feminine and concerned about her appearance at the beginning of the film. She even makes some comments about her daughter's appearance not being feminine enough. As the film progresses and Deborah shifts from source of concern to source of terror (a gothic turn according to Goldman 2017), she is presented as less clean, less proper, and less feminine. Her hair falls out. She is seen in various states of dress and undress. She becomes dirty and bloody. Her skin becomes infected (similar to pressure ulcers). As her body disintegrates, while she is alive, the viewer's sympathies are meant to diminish.

Inability to Care for Homes

In Gothic horror, the physical home is not only a representation of the space itself, but can also represent the psychological state of the individuals that occupy the space (Bailey 1999). In both films, the women's homes belong to them alone and they are not able to take care of them. Each home is in some state of disrepair. Deborah is called a hoarder by her daughter. In each film, there is mention of housing the women in a care facility. In each, the women feel strongly about living in their own homes. But the audience is led to believe that living in their own homes is an irrational or illogical solution, partially because the chaos in the home is meant to represent the failure of the women to remain rational persons.

Inability to Maintain Relationships

A major component of the plot of the films is that the older women are not able to care for themselves. Enter their daughters to help take care of them. In both cases, it is established that neither daughter has a particularly close relationship with their mother. In *Relic*, Edna's potential motherliness is exhibited towards her granddaughter rather than her daughter. An important turn occurs in the narratives of each film. The vulnerable older woman who needs sympathy and care begins to be framed as a source of threat. In *Deborah Logan*, the assumption is that because of her "feeble mind", Deborah is possessed by the ghost of a serial killer. In *Relic*, Edna is possessed by some malevolent entity attached to her home (possibly because her own grandfather was left to die unattended in a shed on her property). The two women violate the expectations of being caregivers. But more troubling is that they violate the expectation that they will be worthy of care. In fact, their mental and physical decline, embodied as the threat that they now pose to the people around them, makes them "unlovable." Being unlovable is the biggest source of failure. Despite being "unlovable", both women are cared for by their daughters Both films make a point to present to the viewer with evidence that neither daughter is close with her mother before the need for caregiving arises, framing the interaction as "duty" (Gouldner 1960 cited in Glenn 2010). In *The Taking of Deborah Logan*, the viewer is given many examples of how Deborah has mistreated Sara in the past. In both films, the decision of the daughter to care for her mother is presented as a burden, something interrupting an already complicated life. Regardless, both daughters in the films consider it their duty to care for their mothers. Both films discussed the status obligation of a daughter to their mother. This duty to the mother is further explored and in *Relic* when Kay and Sam are at the front door finally escaping a monstrous Edna and Kay turns back to care for her mother once more with Sam following behind reluctantly.

Death-in-Life

In *Relic*, Kay embraces her mother's decaying body in the closing scene. She takes great care in removing her mother's skin and hair, revealing her decay. Her actions represent a re-establishing of personhood, a giving back of dignity. That narrative is disrupted however, by Sammie's discovery that her mother Kay is also "infected" with whatever has caused her gran's dementia. It's a brief moment that showcases possibility, and in great horror film fashion, it is taken away.

We argue that ultimately, what we fear when we fear aging is not death. It is partially the seemingly more horrifying notion of death-in-life. Far worse, however, it is the insurmountable distance between our own self and the preferred self of neoliberalism. It is the fear of lack of productivity, and of redundancy. It's the fear of not being lovable enough to be cared for. In recent years, more scholars are investigating how neoliberalism can be resisted at the structural level and also at the level of individual agency, or subjectivity. Work has been examining these counter-hegemonic discourses (Turken et al. 2016). We might offer that what *Relic* and *Deborah Logan* offer is a small space to consider a counter-narrative. Both Edna and Deborah remain cared for by their families, despite no longer sharing their reality, despite not being "loving" "lovable" or "productive". Deborah and Edna had not invested properly in their relationships with their daughters. They had not built enough "care capital" but they still remained valued. Their bodies, their homes, and their persons remain important not to society at large but to their daughters.

Author Bios

Kaydee Corbin Anderson received her master's degree in Sociology from the University of Missouri – Kansas City. She is an Advocate in workforce development for Kansas City Scholars. Her most recent scholarship focuses on the impact of COVID-19 on paid work and care work in the United States. Her academic interests include ageism and film analysis.

Ahoo Tabatabai received her PhD in Sociology from the University of Cincinnati. She is Professor of Sociology at Columbia College in Columbia, Missouri. Her scholarship and teaching interests include the study of narratives and identity. Her work has been published in Disability and Society, Narrative Inquiry, Qualitative Sociology, and Sexualities. She currently serves on the editorial board of Sociological Focus and Social Problems.

Works Cited

Alzheimer's Association, "What is Alzheimer's?," Alzheimer's Disease and Dementia, 2021, https://www.alz.org/alzheimers-dementia/what-is-alzheimers.
Alzheimer's Association, "What is Alzheimer's?," Alzheimer's Disease and Dementia, 2021, https://www.alz.org/alzheimers-dementia/what-is-dementia.
Aquilina, Carmelo and Hughes, Julian, (2006): "The return of the living dead: agency lost and found?" In: Julian C. Hughes/Stephen J. Louw/Steven R. (eds.), Dementia: Mind, Meaning, and the Person, Oxford University Press: Oxford, pp. 143–161.

Bailey, Dale (1999): American Nightmares: The Haunted House Formula in American Popular Fiction, Madison, WI: University of Wisconsin Press.

Ballenger, Jesse F (2006): Self, Senility, and Alzheimer's Disease in Modern America, Baltimore: Johns Hopkins University Press.

Basting, Anne, (2003), "Looking back from loss: views of the self in Alzheimer's disease." Journal of Aging Studies 17, pp. 87–99.

Behuniak, Susan (2011): "The Living Dead? The Construction of People with Alzheimer's Disease as Zombies." Aging & Society 31/1, pp. 70–92.

Black, Hannah (2014): "Crazy in Love." The New Inquiry 35, pp. 8–12.

Butler, Robert. N. (1975.): Why Survive?: Being Old in America. New York: Harper & Row.

Chivers, Sally (2011): "Grey matters: Dementia, Cognitive Difference, and the Guilty Demographic on Screen" in The Silvering Screen: Old Age and Disability in Cinema. University of Toronto Press, Scholarly Publishing Division, pp. 58–74.

Creed, Barbara (1986): "Horror and the Monstrous-Feminine: An Imaginary Abjection." Screen 27/1, pp. 44–71.

Glenn, Evelyn (2010): Forced to Care: Coercion and Caregiving in America, Harvard University Press.

Goffman, Erving (1963): Stigma: Notes on the Management of Spoiled Identity, Touchstone.

Goldman, Marlene (2017): Forgotten: Narratives of Age-Related Dementia and Alzheimer's Disease in Canada, McGill-Queen's University Press.

Haber, Carole (1984): "From Senescence to Senility: The Transformation of Old Age in the Nineteenth Century," International Journal of Aging and Human Development 19, pp. 41–45.

Halberstam, Jack (2011): The Queer Art of Failure, Durham: Duke University Press.

Hantke, Steffen (2007): "Academic Film Criticism, the Rhetoric of Crisis, and the Current State of American Horror Cinema: Thoughts on Canonicity and Academic Anxiety." College Literature. 34/4, pp. 191–202.

Harvey, David (2005): A Brief History of Neoliberalism, Oxford University Press.
Herskovits, Elizabeth (1995): "Struggling over Subjectivity: Debates about the 'Self' and Alzheimer's Disease." Medical Anthropology Quarterly 9 pp. 146–164.
Holstein, M (1997): "Alzheimer's Disease and Senile Dementia, 1885–1920: An interpretive history of disease negotiation." Journal of Aging Studies, 11/1, pp. 1–13.
Hubner, Laura (2018): Fairytale and Gothic Horror: Uncanny Transformations in Film, Palgrave MacMillan.
Jaffe, Sarah (2021): Work Won't Love You Back: How Devotion to Our Jobs Keeps Us Exploited, Exhausted, and Alone, Bold Type Books: New York.
Kawin, Bruce (2012): Horror and Horror Films, New York: Anthem Press.
Luna, Caleb (2018): "Romantic Love Is Killing Us: Who Takes Care of Us When We Are Single?," https://thebodyisnotanapology.com/magazine/romantic-love-is-killing-us/
Matthews, E. (2006): "Dementia and the identity of the person." In: Julian Hughes, Stephen Louw and Steven Sabat. 2006. Dementia: Mind, Meaning, and the Person, International Perspectives in Philosophy and Psychiatry, Oxford: OUP Oxford: pp. 163–178.
McGuigan, Jim (2014): "The Neoliberal Self." Culture Unbound/Journal of Current Cultural Research 6, pp. 223–240.
Miletic, Sasa (2020): "Making a Killing: Norman Bates, Dexter, & Co. as Neoliberal Entrepreneurs of the Self." The Journal of Popular Culture 53/4, pp. 907–925.
Nock, Samantha 2018. "Decrying Desirability: Demanding Care." Guts Magazine. https://www.gutsmagazine.ca.
Norman, Andria/Woodard, John/Calamari, John/Gross, Evan/Pontarelli, Noelle/Socha, Jami/DeJong, Brandon/Kerri Armstrong (2020): "The Fear of Alzheimer's Disease: Mediating Effects of Anxiety on Subjective Memory Complaints." Aging & Mental Health 24/2, pp. 308–314.
Page, Kyle/Hayslip, Bert/Wadsworth, Dee/Allen, Philip (2019): "Development of a Multidimensional Measure to Examine Fear of Demen-

tia." International Journal of Aging and Human Development 89/2, pp. 187–205.

Robertson, Ann. (1991): "The Politics of Alzheimer's Disease: A Case Study in Apocalyptic Demography in Critical Perspectives on Aging." In: Meredith Minkler and C.L. Estes (eds.), The Political and Moral Economy of Growing Old. Amityville, NY: Baywood Publishing Company. pp. 135–150.

Robertson, Laura (2014): "Who Cares?" The New Inquiry Magazine 35, pp. 31–34.

Sabat, Steve and Rom Harré (1992): "The Construction and Deconstruction of Self in Alzheimer's Disease." Aging and Society 12/4, pp. 443–461.

Scheper-Hughes, Nancy and Lock, Margaret (1986): "Speaking Truth to Illness Metaphors, Reification and a Pedagogy for Patients." Medical Anthropology Quarterly 17/5, pp. 137–140.

Shuffelton, Amy (2013): "How Mothers Divide the Apple Pie: Maternal and Civic Thinking in the Age of Neoliberalism." Philosophy of Education Archive, pp. 328–336.

Sontag, Susan (1978): Illness as Metaphor, New York: Farrar.

Stafford, Philip (1991): "The Social Construction of Alzheimer's Disease." In: Sebeok Thomas and Umiker-Sebeok Jean Biosemiotics: The Semiotic Web. (eds.), Berlin: Mouton de Gruyter, pp. 393–406.

Stillman, Sarah (2007): "The Missing White Girl Syndrome: Disappeared Women and Media Activism." Gender and Development 15/3, pp. 491–502.

Turken, Slaman/Hilde Eileen/Nafstad, Rolv/Mikkel Blakar/Katrina Roen (2016): "Making Sense of Neoliberal Subjectivity: A Discourse Analysis of Media Language on Self-development." Globalization 13/1, pp. 32–46.

Villain, Nicolas and Bruno Dubois (2019): "Alzheimer's Disease Including Focal Presentations." Seminars in Neurology 39/2, pp. 213–226.

Wilson, Duncan (2014): "Quantifying the quiet epidemic Diagnosing dementia in late 20th Century Britain." History of the Human Sciences. 5, pp. 126–146.

Zarney, B.D. (June 13, 2021): "Hope and controversy: FDA approves first new Alzheimer's drug in decades." https://www.freethink.com/health/alzheimers-drug-aducanumab

The Southern Slasher Comes of Age
Old Age, Race, and Disability in Ti West's X

Rose Steptoe[1]

This essay considers how Ti West's *X* (2022) reimagines the Southern-set slashers' unique relationship to disability and race through horrific representations of old age. I first discuss *X*'s engagement with *The Texas Chainsaw Massacre* (Hooper, 1974) and argue that slashers set in the American South often indirectly engage histories of racial violence. Southern slashers draw on stereotypes around disability and race to relocate a confrontation with racial violence onto strategically-othered White Southerners, and this is evident in both *X* and *Massacre* through depictions of old age. I then turn to *X* for an analysis of how the film engages tropes from Southern slashers to portray aging in relation to Whiteness, disability, and ultimately, violence. Considering key moments from the film, I conduct an intersectional analysis with relation to age, race, and gender to argue that *X* manipulates and reaffirms the Southern slasher's troubled relationship with disability, where old age in the South has violent implications. Ultimately, *X* builds upon the slasher's longstanding tradition of using coded disability to relocate the histories of racial violence embedded in the Southern slasher. *X* forces us to consider how fears of old age in the slasher are not only connected to physical or mental deterioration, but rather, the inevitability of cyclical violence as time passes with age.

---

1 University of North Carolina at Chapel Hill.

On *The Texas Chainsaw Massacre* and the Legacy of Slashers Set in the American South

While *X* references a variety of independently-produced horror and pornographic films from the 1970s, it most unmistakably evokes the notorious slasher classic, *The Texas Chainsaw Massacre* (Hooper, 1974). One could catalog the many overt, concrete references to Hooper's film in *X* (such as mimicked shot compositions, the protagonists traveling to the house by van, the final girl leaving by pick-up truck, etc.), but the most noteworthy similarity between *X* and *Massacre* is their setting: rural Texas. Rural Texas – and its connotations from Hooper's films extended by West – serves as a geographical reference for socially-construed disability and histories of racial violence. Old age as monstrosity is crafted through *X*'s setting in the American South, and moreover, informed by race: to grow old is to succumb to an urge for barbaric violence, represented through indirect depictions of White supremacist violence in West's film. *X* subverts the typical source of fear in the slasher film: it is not the fear of death, but the fear of surviving – and aging into a monster – that is at the heart of the film's horror. In the first part of this essay, I will consider how *X* plays with *The Texas Chainsaw Massacre*'s presentation of aged Southerners, where White discomfort about race and racial violence is displaced onto the South through representations of disability. As I will discuss in relation to both *Massacre* and *X*, old age functions as a particularly Southern manifestation of disability, where old age is presented as an inevitable social, physical, and moral degradation intrinsic to the landscape.

In *The Texas Chainsaw Massacre*, old age materializes in an extreme and often comedic fashion. In an exemplary scene, the family of cannibalistic slaughterhouse workers sits down for dinner with their victim, Sally (Marilyn Burns). As Robin Wood (1979) has argued, the scene is a distorted parody of a family comedy, where the almost slapstick-like pacing of the sequence follows the younger men in the family encouraging, and then helping, the nearly-dead patriarch of the family ("Grandpa," played by John Dugan) bludgeon Sally in the head. Grandpa's impossibly pale and waxy visage amplifies this physical comedy with the deep-set eyeholes on the mask that Dugan wears – Grandpa looks and moves more like a puppet than a patriarch. Meanwhile, a brief shot in the film also reveals that the family matriarch – "Grandma – is a rotting corpse in the attic, à la Mrs. Bates in *Psycho*. This scene portrays a certain kind of Southern conservatism, evident in an interest in respecting family tradition (Grandpa was the best killer at the slaughterhouse) and maintaining a nuclear, patriarchal family, through absurd, nearly incestuous, and cannibalistic behavior.

Adam Lowenstein argues that Hooper's approach to horror defamiliarizes old age both physically and behaviorally through exaggerated costumes and makeup or by blurring the lines between old and infantile tendencies (2022: 71). With respect to *Massacre*, Lowenstein argues that Grandpa's mix of "babyish" behavior and "impossibly wizened" appearance makes him all-the-more frightening despite his lack of a physical threat (Lowenstein 2022: 79). The film's emphasis on aging is brought to the foreground by Grandpa's constantly transforming relation to his age and feeds on spectatorial fears of liminality by transgressing how we understand age. Lowenstein's analysis of aging, while overall concerned with gender, does not deeply interrogate masculinity in this scene, despite its centrality in characterizing the family's aptly Southern interest in tradition and patriarchy. For example, there is a lack of virility implied by Grandpa's failure to 'finish the job' and deliver a striking blow to Sally's skill. Grandpa's impotence is relevant to his age, and moreover, to this kind of Southern, patriarchal family the scene invokes. While Lowenstein speaks at length about the invisibility experienced by the elderly, his investigation of how gender shapes aging is largely focused on elderly female characters (2022: 75). In doing this, Lowenstein inadvertently construes the male experience of aging as default and assumed, as if men do not have their own unique relationship to aging that is also shaped by their gender. If aging women experience invisibility more than men (Woodward 1999: xiii), then it also seems that in *Texas Chainsaw Massacre*, a masculine relationship to aging is constructed as highly visible, as spectacular, when Grandpa performs (and fails to perform) in front of his family at the dinner table. Meanwhile, Grandma's corpse is hidden away, invisible, and even more impossibly aged, in the attic.

To understand aging in relation to disability, it is crucial to account for how aging is deeply intertwined not only with social constructions of old age, but of gender, and, as I will discuss next, race.

The American South has been a popular venue for slashers to unfold far beyond just *Massacre*. A Southern setting allows for veiled and layered approaches to race and general "otherness" because of the region's fraught past of racial violence and the generalization of its rural character. In this essay, I emphasize the Southern setting, rather than just rural areas, because the Southern geography prevailing in these films ties disability specifically with Southerness and draws on the South's relationship to racial violence to do so. The American South, and more generally rural America, is often described with terms associated with disability, such as "backwards" and "inbred." Moreover, terms of age are ascribed to the region's culture, such as "antiquated." The values of the "Old" South – racism and White supremacy – are perceived as persisting (although not exclusively) in its elderly residents. Critiques of the South invariably invoke notions of disability as impairment, old age as disability, and old age as conservative and even violent. The contradictory assumptions about old age persist throughout Southern-set slashers in complicated ways. For example, what does it mean that having a slasher set in rural Texas can immediately inform how we read the intelligence and cruelty of the characters who live there? Moreover, how can Southerness inform how we consider the social implications of old age in relation to race and disability?

Depictions of the American South in horror films are often rendered visible only through ableist, negative connotations of disability, suggesting that White Southerners are 'inbred' and thus have physical or intellectual differences that inform and exaggerate their "Southerness." This kind of Southern, violent, yet ineffectual monster or killer is a stock character in many horror films. This unintelligent, evil Southerner is so prevalent in slashers that the trope was effectively parodied (and subverted) in the meta-slasher *Tucker and Dale vs. Evil* (Eli Craig, 2011), where two affable "hillbilly" men are mistaken for murderers by a group of teenagers. The film plays with the assumptions of both ignorance and predisposition for violence expected of "backwoods" and "rural" folk in slasher films to great comedic effect. This longstanding association of "hillbillies" with violence has long been replicated even within Southern storytelling, such as in the infamous film adaptation of Georgia author James Dickey's novel *Deliverance*, where a group of Southern, city-dwelling men are terrorized by their more rural counterparts while on a canoeing trip (John Boorman, 1972). Or, to turn even further back in cinematic history to a Southern proto-slasher, one can look to a true "hicksploitation" ("hick" exploitation) film: Herschel Gordon Lewis' *Two Thousand Maniacs!* (1964). Lewis takes Southerners' violence to extremes in his splatter film, where a Southern town celebrates its centennial by torturing and murdering a group of lost road trippers from "the North;" with an all-White cast and a set replete with Confederate flags, its indirect address of White supremacy allowed the film to perform well (if not better than in other regions) on the Southern drive-in circuit (Pinkowitz 2016: 114). But what led to this tradition of evil, White Southerners in the Southern slasher, and why is it so acceptable, if we consider Lewis' film, even to Southerners themselves?

Carol J. Clover, in her influential study of the slasher, makes note of the shift to rural folks as targets for racial anxieties: "If 'redneck' once denoted a real and particular group, it has achieved the status of a kind of universal blame figure, the 'someone else' held responsible for all manner of American social ills. The great success of the redneck in that capacity suggests that anxieties no longer expressible in ethnic or racial terms have become projected onto a safe target – safe not only because it is (nominally) white, but because it is infinitely displaceable onto someone from the deeper South or the higher mountains or the further desert" (Clover 1992: 135). What is underlying 'hicksploitation' horror films and Southern-set slashers, thinly-veiled but rarely engaged directly, is that the brutality associated with Southerness is used to indirectly invoke White supremacist violence. This is largely achieved when White Southerners are depicted as other – through markers of disability – to distinguish them from the protagonist White characters. While Clover describes these White characters as a "safe" target, her argument ignores how Whiteness as a racial category itself is informing the need to make these characters "infinitely displaceable" onto someone more Southern. More Southern, here, means more isolated, less intelligent, more violent, and perhaps physically different in same visible manner. Thus, it is stereotypical markers of disability – both social and physical – used to distance the more urban White victims from the White supremacist associations underlying the violence of the more rural Southerners. The extreme violence of White Southerners in horror films evokes the history of racial violence and lynching of the region while simultaneously masking this history through both an absence of Black characters and any address of race at all

This covert invocation of racial violence in Southern slasher is shaped by a White, liberal "anatomy of guilt," where shame and guilt about racial violence lead to an indirect or symbolic address of the violence, reinforcing ignorance of ongoing racism and histories of racial violence in the South (Crank 2012: 53). The preternaturally violent Southerners in slasher films enact coded racial violence against other White characters (usually from urban areas), and these films neither confront race nor confront the spectator with the truth of the White supremacist violence underlying the film's politics and landscapes. As Richard Dyer discusses, when "white-makings of whiteness" construe Whiteness as the default (as they often do), Whiteness is neither racialized nor acknowledged in what is often called an "invisible" approach to Whiteness (Dyer 1997: xiii). In a film with only White characters, as in many Southern slashers, race is hardly ever addressed at all, even as racism and histories of racial violence undergird the ideologies, geographies, and horrors of these films. Instead, White supremacist attitudes from the region's history are replicated in this neglect of race. bell hooks explains how, "in white supremacist society, white people can 'safely' imagine that they are invisible to black people since the power they have historically asserted...accorded them the right to control the black gaze" (hooks 1998: 41). Just as these films supplant White supremacist violence through representations of disability, they also refuse a Black gaze toward this violence through their displacement of racial violence onto (ableist) conceptions of disability rather than directly confronting race.

By carefully manipulating Whiteness through markers of disability, the Southern slasher has served as a genre where a direct confrontation of race is allayed through violence committed by and against distinctly "other: White characters. Southerners in Southern-set slashers are created as too barbaric, too fundamentally prejudiced, too unintelligent to be identified with by other White characters or White spectators. Rather than directly addressing race, Southern slashers films safely distance these violent Southern killers from Whiteness and the implications of White supremacist violence. In *X*, West picks up, extends, and subverts this trope of White Southerness as "disabled," engaging old age as a form of disability that is particularly Southern in its preoccupation with the past.

Aging the Southern Slasher: Gendered and Racialized Old Age in *X*

Set in 1979, *X* follows a crew of young adults trying to shoot a pornographic film at a farm in rural Texas without the elderly farm owners' knowledge. In *X*, the confluence of the film's Southern geography, an emphasis on Whiteness, and the centrality of old age engages the tropes of the Southern slasher in familiar, reflexive ways. Considering key moments from the film, I will conduct an intersectional analysis with relation to age, gender, and race to continue my argument about Southern slashers and disability. Ultimately, I will argue that *X* manipulates and reaffirms the slasher's troubled relationship with both ageism and disability. Old age in the South means an inevitable return to the past violence embedded in Southern landscapes, resurrected through the passing of time with age.

X is a film with unusually visible elderly characters, and throughout my analysis, I will consider old age through frameworks of ageism and disability. First, I will briefly describe my disability framework. As disability studies scholar Alison Kafer discusses age and disability: "Whether by illness, age, or accident, all of us will live with disability at some point in our lives ... becoming disabled is 'only a matter of time.' Snyder, Brueggemann, and Garland-Thomson call this temporality of inevitability 'the fundamental aspect of human embodiment'" (2013:26).

While aging in relation to disability might be conceived of as a variety of physical or cognitive impairments, there are social models of disability where "disability is socially created through a variety of obstacles that prevent people with impairments from having equal opportunities, access to public spaces, and institutional resources" (Beaudry 2018: 7). For my analysis, I will engage with the socially-inflected aspects of old age to understand age's relationship to other social categories, such as gender and race. As age studies scholar Margaret Gullette notes: "Ageism [is] an ideology based on a master narrative of life-course decline," where older age leads to prejudices that inflect social relationships and various forms of social, economic, and medical support (Gullette 2018: 252). For Gullette, the ageism that accompanies old age is grounded in the social rather than chronological and biological, and ageism's connection to disability is grounded in social hierarchy rather than biological aging. This is not to say the physical elements of aging, which themselves vary greatly due to social factors, are not apt for a disability studies analysis, but rather, that all the various components that comprise the lived experience of old age are can be understood through a social model of what it means to be disabled. It is not impairments themselves that are central to old age as disability, but rather, the ageism faced by elderly people that shapes assumptions and access to resources. My own analysis of X is indebted Gullette's theorization of old age and ageism, as well as to feminist-of-color disability studies, a framework rigorously theorized by Schalk and Kim where race is made a central component of understanding disability in order to "expose 'the ideology of ability in situations that do not appear immediately to be about disability'" (2020: 40).

In X, the "horrors" of old age are conveyed through physical appearance, sexual impotence, and both moral and social decay. The film emphasizes the physical aspects of aging to grotesque extremes meant to repulse the spectator, yet old age is made particularly horrific through the sense of social isolation and attitudes of Pearl and Howard, the film's elderly couple. In the film, aging in the South only means you risk aging into someone resentful, if not violent and prejudiced. Aging as representative of the South's irreparable moral decay is evident even in the film's mise-en-scène, as the couple's dilapidated farmhouse suggests a sense of anachronism and moral deterioration. Perhaps most prominently in X, scenes that trigger fears of what old age means for sexuality capture both the physical and social fears of aging implicit in many Southern-set slashers. Throughout the film, West capitalizes on fears of old age through the juxtaposition of young and old, raising questions of how gender and race are inflected by age, and moreover, using old age's inevitability to create sense of looming violence.

The most pronounced juxtaposition of young and old in X is the mirror image between the film's final girl – the youthful, sexy, and defiant Maxine (Mia Goth) – and its wispy, frail, and desperate killer, Pearl (also Goth, in old age makeup). In having Goth play both characters, the film asks: what does it mean for the final girl to survive? What does it mean for her to age past girlhood and to become in herself a kind of societal monster: an old woman? As Carol J. Clover famously describes, the final girl is the sole survivor at the conclusion of a slasher film – usually young and androgynous, the final girl is tortured and traumatized, yet triumphant over the killer. Implicit in Clover's figure of the final girl and Clover's overall discussion of the slasher film is that the slasher is a genre largely featuring, and made for, teenagers (1992: 35). Age, and particularly youthfulness and its implicit fear of aging, are central to slashers. In X, this relationship between the slasher and aging is encapsulated in Goth's two performances. Goth, 29 years old at the time of filming, is made to appear at an indeterminably old age as Pearl through the remarkable prosthetic and makeup work of Sarah Rubano (Douglas 2022). Rubano transforms Goth beyond recognition – it takes a discerning eye to see that Pearl is indeed played by Goth in makeup. What is readily apparent, however, is that Pearl (and Howard) are made to appear not just old, but grotesque. They have yellowing unkempt hair, an abundance of liver spots, exaggerated eye bags, and teeth in disarray. Pearl and Howard are not inherently frightening because they are old, but rather, they are frightening because they look abandoned and unable to care for themselves. West constructs a purposefully unflattering image of elderly bodies marked by social neglect rather than just old age itself, and this socially-inflected construction of aging is only amplified by the fears of aging divulged by younger characters throughout the film. To return to my claim that old age in the Southern slasher is a continuation of using disability to other White characters, I will examine how the film contrasts young and old through Maxine and Pearl. Maxine is a sexy, young, and confident porn actress. Her outfit – short denim overalls with nothing underneath – evokes the backless shirts and short shorts worn by the female protagonists in *The Texas Chainsaw Massacre*. Maxine takes her youthfulness and open sexuality for granted, with an air of casualness, if not entitlement, to the world – or at least this is how Pearl views her. In the shadows Maxine's brazen sexuality, Pearl reflects back loneliness and desperation. As Katherine Woodward describes how aging pits older women against young: "Younger people (and older people who deny their own aging) have functioned as mirrors to older women, reflecting them back half their size. Surely the practice of the disregard of older women is one of the reasons why in fact we have so many 'little old ladies'" (1999: xii). When Pearl looks at Maxine, she is constructed as the deteriorated version of the younger woman. Not only does this relationship emphasize women's unique experience of aging, but it allows for an understanding of aging in relation to socially-constructed disability. Pearl's social confinement, rather than just physical or cognitive impairments, shapes her ability to navigate the world in old age. She peeks around corners and lurks in the shadows, made not only invisible by society but also socially isolated by virtue of her age. As Gullette describes the social limitations of women's aging, women are more so "aged by culture" than biological aging in itself (Gullette 2004: 6–7). Here, Pearl's frail and frightening appearance exaggerates biological aging, but the film's framing of her behind corners, in shadows, and desperate for connection, illustrate the social constraints of old age that have come to be seen as an implicit part of women's experience of old age. Moreover, Pearl's diminishment in confidence, physical strength, and visibility evoke the child-like passivity often assigned those with disabilities. In Nasa Begum's manifesto for women with disabilities, she describes: "Stereotypes of passivity and childlike dependency are created for members of the 'disabled' and, at the same time, roles are prescribed which render us powerless" (1992: 71). Pearl embodies the chronological contradiction described by Begum: she is old yet childlike, passive yet also later, violent. This anachronism is particularly apt for Southern slasher as it replicates the South's own obsession with the past in the present.

West juxtaposes the youthfulness of the porn industry (Maxine) with the old age that presupposes the source of violence of in the horror film (Pearl). In porn, the spectator is meant to unabashedly look, while horror aims for a spectator to look away; throughout X, Maxine and Pearl's relationship is negotiated looking toward and away from each other. This looking is not just a reference to woman-as-spectacle-object – as porn star, final girl, or monster – but also a form of looking forward and back in time. The glances the women exchange throughout the film are ones of looking back at the past and forward to the future. It is a relationship of contrast between visibility and invisibility, between leering in sexual desire and looking on in horror. Maxine catches Pearl from around a corner, a window, peeking out – Maxine must effort to see Pearl, and when she does, she's frightened. In contrast, Pearl capitalizes on the connection between youthful sexuality, femininity, and hypervisibility, voyeuring Maxine as she skinny dips and Maxine performs while shooting the crew's pornographic film. Pearl's gaze is one of both a desire to be seen like Maxine, and to be with Maxine. Pearl's sexual repression and desire manifest in her look at Maxine, and when this desire is not met, Pearl's frustration turns to aggression and explosive violence as she begins to murder the pornography crew. Indeed, Pearl's lack of access to sex is where Pearl resents Maxine the most. At the film's violent conclusion, Pearl states what she and Maxine both fear the most: "We're the same. You'll end up just like me." To become "just like" Pearl is to become invisible, to lose sexual desirability, and, to be driven to violence. As feminist age studies scholars have noted, a key aspect of women's experience of aging is how they are made invisible, and inherent in this invisibility is the loss of heterosexual desirability (Woodward 1999: xiii),

The presentation of Pearl's old age, and experience of age as disability, is necessarily informed by notions of White femininity, where Pearl's frailty and childlike helplessness are presented as a universal experience of old age. Pearl's femininity and initial weakness, while shaped by ageism, reinforce White femininity as docile and a universal experience of old age. The racialized implications of Pearl's femininity in relation to aging can be bolstered when contrasted with a reading of Black women's experience of disability. As Bailey and Mobley note: "The myth of the strong Black woman ... suggests that Black women are uniquely strong, able to endure pain, and surmount otherwise difficult obstacles because of their innate tenacity. Black women are disallowed disability and their survival is depoliticized" (2019: 21). Whereas Black women are not granted weakness, White women's experience of age calls for a kind of frailty that acts as an exaggerated version of White femininity's demure docility. This relationship to old age, particularly in relation to invisibility and weakness, is part of a larger White supremacist framework that enforces White women's "need" to be protected. Schalk and Kim, in their feminist-of-color critique of disability studies, describe how "Discourses of (dis)ability...have been used to create, maintain, and justify racial and gender hierarchies (and the various injustices and violence that result from such hierarchies) in numerous ways across various historical moments" (2020: 40). Here, too, expectations for White women's femininity, when confronted with old age, can be used to uphold White supremacist constructions of femininity, even when informed by disability. This social consideration of the ageism informing Pearl's supposed frailty places her violence later in the film in the context of larger histories of violence and disability in Southern slashers.

The other half of *X*'s elderly homicidal couple, Howard (Stephen Ure), provides further nuance to questions of aging, gender, and race in the film. In Howard, the film's engagement with the Southern slasher's complex relationship to race becomes more overt: *X* reinforces the South as a setting that can be used to invoke racial anxiety and a connection between old age and White supremacist ideology. Whereas Pearl and Maxine are doubled, an embodiment of past and present captured by Mia Goth, Howard's age is thrown into relief by someone different than him. Howard develops a tenuous working relationship with one of the porn actors, the young, Black, and (perhaps stereotypically) virile Jackson Hole (Kid Cudi). Howard and Jackson are framed as foils early in the film. While never explicitly stated, racial tension underlies the scenes with Howard and Jackson, where an elderly, White, Southern man and a young Black man are placed in unfamiliar situations together. Moreover, these men are constructed as opposites in relation to their sexual virility. A humorous gag shot of Jackson Hole's nude shadow portrays him as physically well-endowed; in contrast, Howard constantly refuses Pearl's sexual advances because of his weak heart. This difference is furthered through their respective sexual encounters in the film: Jackson is energetic in the crew's pornographic film, while Howard's sex scene, framed within a long, bird's-eye shot, only makes him appear even more vulnerable. At first, the film plays with the tension between Howard and Jackson, teasing an almost saccharine relationship arc when the two bond over both having served in the military. Yet, the differences between the two men prevail, confirming spectatorial expectations embedded in cinematic tropes around race; as the two walk through a dark bayou, Howard shoots Jackson in the back with seemingly no motivation. Howard's murder of Jackson affirms spectatorial fears introduced when the first two met – a fear of racial violence between a presumably prejudiced older White man and a young Black man. Howard's resentment of Jackson's sexual virility is inflected with both racial stereotypes affirmed by the film and the kind of racism stereotypically associated with older, particularly Southern, White men. While Pearl resents Maxine for embodying what she could have been, Howard resents Jackson for everything he is not. X rehearses the rhetoric of the Southern slasher where race is never directly addressed yet underlies the ideologies underlying the film's violence.

In its pastiche approach, X exploits and affirms the Southern slasher as a venue for addressing the fear of aging as a fear of "old" values. The film makes old age's potential loss of sexuality hypervisible and grotesque, but also an inevitability. Between Maxine and Pearl, horror and pornography's longstanding connection is constructed as an evolution from the youthfulness and sexual desirability apparent in pornography to the supposed horrors of being an old woman. In a reconfiguration of *The Texas Chainsaw Massacre*, X concludes with Maxine driving a pick-up truck away from the farm, refusing to look back.

However, in refusing to see and acknowledge Pearl – to look back to her possible future – Maxine inscribes her own fate. As the surviving final girl, Maxine entrusts the inevitability of her own aging. X reconfigures the final girl's relationship to her sexuality as doomed precisely because she survives. Maxine's youthfulness and sexuality are not punished by death, as they would be in a typical slasher from the 1970s and 1980s; rather, her punishment is surviving, living on to age, and risking "ending up" just like Pearl.

In X, aging is not a forward progression, but rather, an inescapable cycle. The cyclical nature of aging, as a marker of disability and indicator of impending violence, alludes to the cycles of racial violence embedded in Southern landscapes, as well as the cyclical nature of violence in slashers as a genre. Given the inevitability of aging, X's Southern setting reaffirms the connection between Southern slashers and disability. X unselfconsciously uses aging as a new means of invoking disability, continuing to avoid an explicit engagement with the histories of racial violence that inform Southern slashers. Analyzing old age alongside notions of disability and race, as I have done throughout this essay, forces us to carefully reconsider how and why old age appears in horror films. Horror films hardly ever just present a fear of chronological, biological aging. Rather, old age in the horror film, when complicated by gender, race, and disability, reveals much greater social anxieties about past injustices inevitably, and violently, reemerging through the passing of time.

Author Bio

Rose Steptoe is a Ph.D. Candidate in English and Comparative Literature at the University of North Carolina at Chapel Hill. Her dissertation focuses on the intersection of feminist film theory and body horror, and more broadly, she is interested in horror's capacity to engage questions of gender and sexuality across disparate aesthetic and generic formulations.

Works Cited

Bailey, Moya, & Mobley, Izetta Autumn (2019): "Work in the Intersections: A Black Feminist Disability Framework." *Gender & Society*, 33(1), 19–40. https://doi.org/10.1177/0891243218801523.

Beaudry, Jonas-Sébastien (2018): "Theoretical Strategies to Define Disability," in Adam Cureton, and David T. Wasserman (eds.), *The Oxford Handbook of Philosophy and Disability*, New York: Oxford University Press.

Begum, Nasa (1992): "Disabled Women and the Feminist Agenda." *Feminist Review*, no. 40, 70–84. https://doi.org/10.2307/1395278.

Clover, Carol J. (1992): *Men, Women, and Chainsaws: Gender in the Modern Horror Film*. Princeton, N.J.: Princeton University Press.

Crank, James A (2012): "Racial violence, receding bodies: James Agee's anatomy of guilt." in Lofaro, M. (Ed.): *Agee at 100: Centennial essays on the works of James Agee*. Knoxville: University of Tennessee Press.

Douglas, Edward (2022): "X Hair and Makeup Designer Sarah Rubano on Turning Mia Goth Into Pearl and Working With Ti West." in *Below the Line*, April 20 (https://www.btlnews.com/crafts/sarah-rubano-x-movie-pearl-hair-makeup-interview/).

Dyer, Richard (1997): *White: Essays on race and culture*. London and New York: Routledge.

Gullette, Margaret Morganroth (2004): *Aged by Culture*. Chicago: University of Chicago Press.

Gullette, Margaret Morganroth (2018): "Against 'Aging'– How to Talk about Growing Older." *Theory, Culture & Society*, 35(7–8), 251–270. https://doi.org/10.1177/0263276418811034.

hooks, bell. "Representations of Whiteness in the Black Imagination" pp. 38–84 in Roediger, David R., ed. (1998): *Black on White: Black Writers on What It Means to Be White*. 1st ed. New York: Schocken Books.

Kafer, Alison (2013): *Feminist, Queer, Crip*. Bloomington, Indiana: Indiana University Press.

Lowenstein, Adam (2022): *Horror Film and Otherness*, New York: Columbia University Press.

Pinkowitz, Jacqueline (2016): "Down South: Regional Exploitation Films, Southern Audiences, and Hillbilly Horror in Herschell Gordon Lewis's Two Thousand Maniacs!(1964)," *Journal of Popular Film and Television*, 44:2, pp. 109–119, https://doi.org/10.1080/01956051.2015.1089831.

Schalk, Sami, and Jina B. Kim (2020): "Integrating Race, Transforming Feminist Disability Studies." *Signs: Journal of Women in Culture and Society* 46, no. 1: 31–55. https://doi.org/10.1086/709213.

Wood, Robin (2018 [1979]): "The American Family Comedy: From Meet Me in St. Louis to The Texas Chainsaw Massacre" (1979). In *Robin Wood on the Horror Film: Collected Essays and Reviews*, edited by Barry Keith Grant. Detroit, Michigan: Wayne State University Press.

Woodward, Kathleen (1999): "Introduction" in Kathleen Woodward (ed.). *Figuring Age: Women, Bodies, Generations*. Bloomington: Indiana University Press, pp. ix-xxix.

"With Strange Aeons Even Death May Die"
Aging in the World of Cthulhu

Joel Soares Oliveira[1]

Lovecraft's presence in the horror genre is ever increasing and his influence is discernible in every artistic medium. We find references to his works in books, films, comic books, videogames and even music. He is the central figure of the genre we often call "weird fiction"; with it appears the term "cosmic horror", that is often used to categorize various works of art that take as a theme or problem the ideas that were put forward by Lovecraft so many years in the past. Even so, of all the themes and images that we find in his short stories, his monsters are still his best-known creations. We all have read or heard about Cthulhu and many other beings that with him make up the mythos of Lovecraftian horror, and these creatures are the focus of this chapter.

These monsters do not share that many characteristics with one another: the lack of a comprehensive description and the agglomeration of adjectives are what make the tales of this author so effective at provoking terror in the reader. The literary techniques that create these creatures of the unknown will be discussed further below, but for now I want to make clear one of the proprieties that is common to most of them: their completely different apprehension of time compared to human beings. With this what I want to emphasize is the fact that Cthulhu, for example, experiences time in a way that is closer to the geological time of earth, which is measured in increments of thousands of years; such a scale is totally foreign to the human mind, that which counts the passing of time

---

1   University of Porto.

in weeks, years and, at limit, centuries. This discrepancy between the human time and the time of the "Old Ones" is important, and it is the cause of our own inability to fully comprehend geological changes and climate change. The overlap between geological time and the time of these creatures is a crucial point for the topics that will be discussed in this essay.

Kathleen Woodward, in her article "Ageing in the Anthropocene: The View From and Beyond Margaret Drabble's *The Dark Flood Rises*" (2020), points out that in Drabble's novel the "collision of ordinary human time experienced in terms of the orderly expectations of middle-class life regarding longevity (as phobic as the fourth age might be regarded), with the longue durée of geological time, time punctuated by inevitable if unpredictable large-scale catastrophe" (Woodward 2020: 50). Throughout her essay, the author explores the relation between human aging and the geological time that surpasses it, how the second can help us understand the first and vice-versa: the way we understand our own aging, be it positively or negatively, is put into perspective when compared to geological time, in which the average human life has no real consequence. In this perspective, when comparing a human life to the scale of geological time, in which a million of years is not that long, our perception of our own place in the universe is undermined and we suddenly appear meaningless. As we try to understand such changes that happen in the time span of the earth, we eventually ask ourselves what "old" really means, as well as what makes someone old, when we are but a speck in the countless years that have gone by since the planet was formed. I want to take these ideas as a starting point for this chapter, substituting geological time for the "Old Ones" time as a measure for our own time; in other words, to challenge mainstream notions of aging and what that entails, juxtaposing them to the incomprehensible life of these fantastic beings that have existed for millions of years and will surely be around after human have become extinct.

Is worth mentioning at this point the concept of "deep time", alluded to since the beginning, but not in an explicit fashion. "Deep time" refers to the temporal scale of geological alterations, natural disasters, climate change and the "Old Ones". At this scale, time is measured in thousands of years, millions of years, in which a century, a decade, a human life are nothing more but a brief moment in the history of deep time. Such large periods of time are effectively unthinkable for the human mind. Human thought perceives the passing of time in years, centuries or even as generations, the latter concept allowing us to travel further into the past and into the future. Compare this to "deep time", an idea of time in which changes are slow, imperceptible to the human eye and difficult to understand. Cthulhu clearly belongs to "deep time", since not only does he live in a way that is impossible for us to fathom, but also it is this impossibility that gives him his mystique as a character from a horror tale: as we will see, the omnipresent characteristic in every Lovecraftian creation is its total resistance to human thought. A brief excerpt from Helen Gordon (2021) can help us understand this:

> Geologists, I was beginning to realise, see the world a little differently from other people. It comes from living half inside what we might call human time and half inside another larger, weirder scale – that of deep time. If human time is measured in seconds and minutes, hours and years, then deep time deals with hundreds of thousands of years, with the millions and the billions. Thinking about it engenders a sort of temporal vertigo. To live in deep time is to take the long view, which means getting your head into a somewhat different place. In deep time it is not just what happened last week or last year or last decade that matters – it's also what happened a million, 50 million, 500 million years ago. It's about the ways in which the succession of events across those millions of years can be said to explain why you're here right now in this particular place, in this particular moment. (Gordon 2021: 1)

And we can also look at an excerpt from the short story "Dagon" that demonstrates how these themes are present in the works of Lovecraft:

> Through some unprecedented volcanic upheaval, a portion of the ocean floor must have been thrown to the surface, exposing regions which for innumerable millions of years had lain hidden under unfathomable watery depths. (Lovecraft 2002: 2)

These themes are a staple of the style and horror of Lovecraft, they come up, for that reason, in other works of literature made in the universe of this author, as we can see in the next excerpt from the book *Sherlock Holmes and the Shadwell Shadows* (2016) from the series Cthulhu Casebooks by James Lovegrove:

> The chieftain laughed balefully. 'They are not the infants. We are. The gods are old, 'older than time. They came here from the stars, from other worlds, while the Earth was still young and unformed.' (Lovegrove 2016: 217)

While most readers will likely know what climate change is and what it entails, even if only by being witness to its effects these last few years, the same cannot be said for the works and monsters of Lovecraft. Because of that, it seems prudent to briefly explore these creatures, their characteristics, and astonishing dimensions, in a way that we can better understand where they stand vis-a-vis the discussion of aging that we are trying to study.

Lovecraft's monsters defy the parameters between what is living and what is dead: these monsters either seem like they do not die, or they are dead and alive at the same time, and in some cases may not even have ever been alive in the first place. Even the word "monster" that is frequently used when talking about these topics can be deceiving. We have a preconceived image of what a monster is. The power of Lovecraft's creation lies in the total undefinition of the beings we are told about. This is best observed in the lacking descriptions the narrators make in all the stories: the monstrous is in the unknowable.

These creatures are terror-inducing because they are unknown; seeing such beings reveals to the watcher the limits of her own thought. The revelation of such a limitation of thought is what drives the characters to madness. Eugene Thacker says the following about this topic:

> The threat is not the monster, or that which threatens existing categories of knowledge. Rather, it is the "nameless thing," or that which presents itself as a horizon for thought. If the monster is that which

cannot be controlled (the unlawful life), then the nameless thing is that which cannot be thought (the unthinkable life). Why can it not be thought? Not because it is something unknown or not- yet known (the mystical or the scientific). Rather, it is because it presents the possibility of a logic of life, though an inaccessible logic, one that is absolutely inaccessible to the human, the natural, the earthly – an "entelechy of the weird." (Thacker 2010: 23)

This resonates with what Lovecraf himself says at the beginning of his best-known story, "The Call of Cthulhu":

The most merciful thing in the world, I think, is the inability of the human mind to correlate all its contents. We live on a placid Island of ignorance in the midst of black seas of infinity, and it was not meant that we should voyage far. The sciences, each straining in tis own direction, have hitherto harmed us little; but some day the piecing together of dissociated knowledge will open up such terrifying vistas of reality, and of our frightful position therein, that we shall either go mad from the revelation or flee from the deadly light into the peace and safety of a new dark age. (Lovecraft 2002: 139)

We find a tension between the attempt to classify these beings, beginning with calling them "old ones" even though we cannot really know how old they are or when they were born, and ending with the multiple descriptions that use abundant adjectives that are never enough or helpful to paint the picture of what the character is seeing.

To really understand how Lovecraft conveys to his reader this unthinkable nature of his creatures, we must first look at his literary style and how his characters narrate what happens around them. One facet of his writing, and really of most horror literature (which he accentuates), is the creation of suspense by means of hiding or giving the least possible amount of information about the monster that is trying to scare us. Throughout the stories we are given glimpses of the nature of the being we should fear; the lack of information builds tension, and the monster ends up being more frightening than it would have been if described right at the beginning or at first sight. Here we must clarify that, even though this is common in most horror media, Lovecraft takes it one step further, making his descriptions extremely cryptic, since his creations are not meant to be understood, or described for that matter.

Therefore, when the protagonist describes finally what he has seen, we get only a very brief one at that, intentionally. In those descriptions there is a constant tension between the being that the narrator is seeing and that is real, and what the narrator can actually tell us about it. Graham Harman points to two important characteristics in Lovecraft's style that cause this difficulty in understanding completely what is being described:

> This is the stylistic world of H.P. Lovecraft, a world in which (1) real objects are locked in impossible tension with the crippled descriptive powers of language, and (2) visible objects display unbearable seismic torsion with their own qualities. (Harman 2012: 36)

So, Harman finds these two facets of the author's style. On one hand, there is the constant limitation of the language itself and the necessary tools to describe the beings that appear in these stories; sometimes the narrator will identify and express this difficulty he has in finding the right words or phrases to tell us what he is seeing. On the other hand, we notice a collision between the empirical and real object observed by a subject and the attempt to enumerate his various qualities, this, contrary to what we would expect, makes everything even more confusing. The focus of the description continues illogically unrecognizable and the various qualities that are given to it appear to not connect between themselves. We are left with a paradoxical image in our minds as we read these texts.[2]

---

2   We have here an example of this from "The Call of Cthulhu": "Above the apparent hieroglyphics was a figure of evidently pictorial intent, though its impressionistic execution forbade a very clear idea of its nature. It seemed to be a sort of monster, or symbol representing a monster, of a form which only a diseased fancy could conceive. If I say that my somewhat extravagant imagination yielded simultaneous pictures of an octopus, a dragon, and a human caricature, I shall not be unfaithful to the grotesque and scaly body with rudi-

It is the author's own style that exacerbates the impossibility of these and let us experience indirectly the panic and existential crisis lived by the characters in his tales. Again, it's in this that that we find the true terror of his works, the horror of revelation, when human reasoning finds something that goes beyond reason and logic as is known to it; the human race is then moved from the top of the animal world to lower in the scale: his own intellectual capability that secured the top spot above all other known animals is confronted with its limits.

We should note that in some cases even a description is too much. We can find instances where Lovecraft gives us a name, foreign to our known names of course, and we are given not a single description of what that name might be attached to. The most we get is some sound, color or object that hints at the being, but other than that is total unknown.

Despite belonging to the domain of "strange fiction", his style and narratives are different from what was standardized for the genre at the time. The stories that were commonly published in the various "pulp magazines" had the typical monsters we are used to seeing and protagonists who were not surprised by their existence.[3] But here the protagonists exacerbate the effect of the terror caused by the various monsters through their reaction as they first lay eyes on them. They react in the same way as any reader would when faced with such a creature:

---

mentary wings; but it was the *general outline* of the whole witch made it most shockingly frightful. Behind the figure was a vague suggestion of Cyclopean architectural background." (Lovecraft 2002: 141).

3   Some examples of this: "Instintively, by a sort of sub-concious preparation, he kept himself and his forces well in hand the whole evening, compelling an accumulative reserve of control by that nameless inward process of gradually putting all the emotions away and turning the key upon them – a process difficult to describe, but wonderfully effective" (Blackwood 2014: 2929); "But her face he never properly saw. A muffler of white fur buried her neck to the ears, and her cap came over the eyes. He only saw that she was young. Nor could he gather her hotel or chalet, for she pointed vaguely, when he asked her, up the slopes. 'Just over there-' she said, quickly taking his hand again. He did not press her; no doubt she wished to hide her escapade" (Blackwood 2014: 2865).

terrified, paralyzed and, most of the time, maddened. This reaction also plays an important role in the desired effect of the horror tale.

Going back to the idea of "deep time" that we discussed earlier, the temporal scale of the monsters also plays an important role in how terrifying they are. These are beings that live in a chronology totally different from that of the human being, so different that it becomes inconceivable for the human mind to think or imagine ages so much earlier than its own. It is again the terror of the unknown and the unthinkable, this time in temporal terms: there is the realization that humanity is a very small chapter in the history of the universe, that these beings have a totally different experience from ours and we will never understand it, hence the terror when discovering ancient ruins or artifacts from civilizations that surpass us, as they become, like the monsters, beyond our logical and intellectual capacity, and this difficulty in placing them in a timeline is what creates terror.

Let's look at some examples and start with the fish-men from *The Shadow Over Innsmouth*. The terror of this story is linked, in addition to the monsters we find in it, to the revelation of the origins of the small town, its relationship with strange aquatic beings and the protagonist's discovery, at the end of the narrative, that he himself is a descendant of that " species". These fish-men show strange characteristics, in their skin, in their eyes, in the sounds they produce, which become more and more marked with age,[4] until these fish-men reach a stage of development in which they become completely aquatic and practically immortal, joining the other aquatic beings, which only the protagonist has heard of, living from then on in the ocean. This latest information comes from the city drunk, which we can see below, although it is not very clear:

---

4   "Rough and scabby, and the sides of their necks are all shriveled or creased up. Get bald, too, very young. The older fellows look the worst – fact is, I don't believe I've ever seen a very old chap of that kind. Guess they must die of looking into the glass! Animals hate'em – they used to have lots of horse trouble before autos came in."; "His age as perhaps thirty-five, but the odd, deep creases in the side of his neck made him seem older when one did not study his dull, expressionless face.", (Lovecraft 2002: 273);

> When it come to matin' with them toad-lookin' fishes, the Kanakys kind of balked, but finally they learnt something as put a new face on the matter. Seems that human folks has got a kind o' relation to sech water-beasts – that everything alive come out on the water once, an' only needs a little change to go back again. Them things told the Kanakys that ef they mixed bloods there's be children as ud look human at fust, but later turn more 'n more like the things, till finally they'd take to the water an' jine the main lot o' things down thar. An' this is the important part, young feller – them as turned into fish things an' went into the water couldn't die. Them things never died excep' they was kilt violent. (Lovecraft 2002: 297)

This type of evolution we see in the Innsmouth fish-men certainly raises questions about how we view aging. These beings are discriminated against for their appearance and their apparent degradation over the years, not very different from what we might associate with human beings. However, this loss of capabilities that is taking place is not a complete loss for the subject, rather a stage that prepares you for a new life underwater. To a certain extent we cannot speak here of premature aging, after all these fish-men will have a long life; their journey on land could even be seen as the equivalent of childhood in another species. This is interesting also when drawing a parallel between these beings that evolve in a strange way to adapt to an aquatic environment and the living beings that first started adapting to live on land and began the evolution that made us humans today. Again, this questions what it is actually ageing and how different ways of aging are not bad by default.

Cynthia Port, in her essay "No Future: Aging, Temporality, History, and Chronologies" (2012), explores how culture, politics and society view older people and, by contrast, younger people. Throughout her text, she highlights the tendency for neo-liberal societies to devalue the elderly by overvaluing the youngest. The discourse is already known, the youngest are the future, they will be useful and productive, while the elderly are seen as useless and, in a way, without a future. It's clearly a negative view of aging; as we age, we move towards uselessness. In this view, Innsmouth poses a major problem for Port, as aging is clearly a loss of capacities that impede participation in human society. However, it would be argued that it is not exactly a loss, it would rather be a transformation, these beings are now able to carry out new tasks, and perhaps even more effectively, only in a non-human society. The challenge posed by the tale to our conception of aging is evident: growing old will not be a path of loss and uselessness, it is a transformation, it is an exchange of physical capacities, in the case of human beings, for others that will not be less valuable.

And, remembering "deep time" again, the precocious aging that the beings of Innsmouth show is only precocious from a human point of view. In reality, they also pose a challenge to the way we experience time: people from Innsmouth will live much longer than any human being,[5] hence the characterization as precocious demonstrates the anthropocentric view we have of aging.

The "Old Ones" are also quite interesting when it comes to the discussion of aging. It should be clarified that this classification is not exactly rigid, so to simplify things, when we speak of "Old Ones" we're referring to all those beings that existed long before humanity, who surpass their capacity for thought, not being possible to place them among living or non-living beings in the formerly spoken conception, as, for instance, Cthulhu and Nyarlathotep.

They are beings that live in a chronology totally different from the human one, that of "deep time", and they are clearly a type of life totally different from what we conceive: they do not die, they do not age, as far as we can know, and they defy the natural laws we are accustomed to. The fear they cause us is the same that Woodward attributes to climate change; both the "Old Ones" and climate change belong to "deep time", their actions are slow and comprise periods of time that are totally unthinkable to us, and it is this fact that makes these creatures so terrifying, because, as we already mentioned above, they place themselves beyond the human intellect and thought.

---

5   "Folks as had took to the water gen'rally come back a good deal to visit, so's a man ud often be a-talkin' to his own five-times-great-grandfather, who'd left the dry land a couple o'hundred years or so afore." (Lovecraft 2002: 298).

Helen Small studies how the way we see age, how we experience it, is dependent on the culture in which we find ourselves. Stereotypes change, like any cultural phenomenon, but Small also claims that age is a subjective and relative experience. Each one will necessarily have a way of seeing aging, a way of experiencing it and acting it, or acting out their age; but beyond that, our age is flexible, we feel younger when we interact with someone who is older, and the opposite is also true, when in the presence of someone younger, we feel the opposite. Evidently aging is experienced mainly according to prejudices. Furthermore, our assumptions about old age are actually paradoxical:

> For every conventional negative association of 'old age' there is an equally recognizable counter-association: rage/serenity; nostalgia/detachment; folly/wisdom; fear/courage; loss of sexual powers and/or opportunities/liberation from sex; loss of the capacity or right to labour/release from a long life of labour. (Small 2007: 27)

This reinforces the idea that aging is not simply a loss of capabilities. Even if we do lose some physical attributes, which is normal as the body ages, we also gain new tools and attributes, mainly psychological, that help us participate in different tasks, ones that are still important for society. In a way, Small shows us that aging is very much guided by sociological and cultural forces, not entirely biology.[6]

---

6   It is interesting to point out here that old people in the tales of Lovecraft present more positive qualities attributed to old age, than negatives. We have various examples: the old man in *The Shadow over Innsmouth* may have seen better days when it comes to being sober and healthier, but he is above all else a wise man, who is presented as the only connection the protagonist can have with the past and the history of the town. In *The Dreams in the Witch House*, we can find something similar. The old woman is represented as powerful and cunning, in contrast with the oblivious protagonist. These examples can briefly show how Lovecraft tends to portray older people, and older beings in general, as more knowledgeable, and capable in certain scenarios. In his works, the loss of physical capabilities is often counterbalanced by mainly positive stereotypes about old age.

These stereotypes aren't only a way to see and judge others, it also guides our behavior. Complementing the work of Small, Mary Russo, in her article "Aging and the Scandal of Anachronism" (1999), tries to show how these assumptions play a big part in the way we act and expect others to act. She argues that we maintain an idea of chronological aging, where each moment of our life comprises some activities that we can or cannot perform, certain characteristics that we must incorporate; aging is gradual and entails changes in our behavior, culturally defined, which imply an evolution, which, on the contrary, obliges us to avoid behaviors that are prior to our age, or after it. Russo then talks about a phenomenon she calls anachronism, which in this context refers to the moment when a certain subject acts "incorrectly" for his age. The effect of anachronism is mostly social, just as the social dictates what is right, an act of anachronism will be met with criticism and ridicule.

The "Old Ones", following these two theorists, lead to two interesting ideas. The first is the difficulty they offer to understanding their own aging: a human subject will never understand how old one of these beings will be, the name "Old Ones" that is used to group them is clearly fallacious, it is a nomenclature with anthropocentric point of reference, however, the use of the word "old" is generally pejorative when we talk about living beings, but here it seems to reinforce the idea that their temporal experience is totally different from ours. "Old" seems to group much more of the positive prejudices that we associate with old age, as Helen Small suggests. The second and more interesting idea is how we can relate our age to such beings. We discussed above how we often view our age subjectively and in comparison, to those around us. Following this reasoning, the presence and revelation of the "Old Ones" creates a certain compression effect on the longevity of human life, which suddenly seems shorter. A young person and an elderly person, when compared to these "deep time" beings, are very close; for such beings they are clearly indistinguishable, which in the various tales is one of the horror aspects for the characters, which does not fail to raise questions about the distinctions we make based on age.

This essay only presents some ideas in this link between aging studies and Lovecraft's work. There is still a lot to explore in theoretical terms, and we only touched on a few short stories in passing, which is an injustice to them, as each one deserved a text on the subject. I think it was possible, even so, to see that these creatures that appear in the narratives create interesting problems in the way we think and conceptualize aging itself, historically thought from a human perspective, and simultaneously create tensions that allow us to better understand ourselves as humans.

Author Bio

Joel Soares Oliveira holds an MA in Literary, Culture and Interartistic Studies from the University of Porto. In 2023, he defended his MA thesis, titled "Religions of the Future: Tensions and Confluences between Religion and Science in SF Novels by Robert Zelazny, Frank Herbert and Neil Stephenson.

Works Cited

Blackwood, Algernon (2014): The Works of Algernon Blackwood, Delphi Classics.
Gordon, Helen (2021): Notes from Deep Time: A Journey Through Our Past and Future Worlds, London, Profile Books.
Harman, Graham (2012): Weird Realism: Lovecraft and Philosophy, Winchester, Zero Books.
Lovecraft, H. P. (2002): The Call of Cthulhu and Other Weird Stories, London, Penguin Classics.
Lovecraft, H. P. (2002): The Dreams in the Witch House and Other Weird Stories, London, Penguin Classics.
Lovecraft, H. P. (2002): The Thing in the Doorstep and Other Weird Stories, London, Penguin Classics.
Lovegrove, James (2016): Sherlock Holmes and the Shadwell Shadows, London, Titan Books.

Port, Cynthia (2012): "No Future: Aging, Temporality, History, and Chronologies" In: Occasion IV.

Russo, Mary (1999): "Aging and the Scandal of Anachronism" In: Figuring Age: Women, Bodies, Generations, pp. 20.33.

Small, Helen (2007): The Long Life, Oxford, Oxford University Press.

Thacker, Eugene (2010): After Life, Chicago, University of Chicago Press.

Woodward, Kathleen (2020): "Aging in the Anthropocene; The View From and Beyond Margarest Drabble's The Dark Flood Rises" In: Literature and Ageing, pp. 37–63.

"And I'm Going to Get Old"
Age Horror in the *Twilight* Franchise[1]

Ruth Gehrmann[2]

Twilight, Horror and Non-Aging

Engaging with *The Twilight Saga*[3] in an edition subtitled *Old Age in Horror Fiction and Film* draws a connection that might cause offense. After all, many invested in the genre of horror have gone through great lengths to emphasize that Stephenie Meyer's novels (2005–2020)[4] and the films (2008–2012) they inspired are not to be considered horror. For instance, in 2009 a blog post on *Twilight Sucks* emotionally explains: "Vampires use

---

1   This article is based on research developed in the Collaborative Research Center 1482 "Human Differentiation," which is funded by the German Research Foundation (DFG), and which is based at Johannes Gutenberg-University Mainz, Germany. I am also indebted to my colleagues at the Obama Institute for Transnational American Studies at Johannes Gutenberg-University Mainz, Germany for their thoughtful comments and insights.
2   Johannes Gutenberg-University Mainz.
3   In the following, *Twilight* is used to refer to the franchise as a whole. When I refer to the series' first installment of the same name, I will specifically address it.
4   Stephenie Meyer has published a variety of publications set in the *Twilight* universe, including the novella *The Short Second Life of Bree Tanner* (2010), *Life and Death* (2015), in which Bella and Edward swap genders, and *Midnight Sun* (2020), a retelling of *Twilight* from Edward's perspective. In this article, I focus on the four key novels of what has been termed *The Twilight Saga*: *Twilight* (2005), *New Moon* (2006), *Eclipse* (2007) and *Breaking Dawn* (2008) as well as their adaptations to film.

[sic] to be a cult-following, much like how anime use [sic] to be in the West. Now, it's everywhere, and has lost its meaning. I weep for literature, the underground subcultures, and humanity as a whole for accepting this book with praise" (spirt_mage_234 2009). The quote – and the frustration it expresses – emphasizes a shift from the margins to the center: *Twilight* has amassed a following, drawing attention not only at box offices and book sales but also in fan clubs and conventions,[5] thus being anything but *niche*. In fact, *Twilight* has moved beyond being a successful series of young adult fiction and has become a household name and a multimillion-dollar franchise.

The story follows first-person narrator Isabella (Bella) Swan's love-triangle with shapeshifter Jacob Black and vampire Edward Cullen and ends with her not only marrying and having a child with the latter but becoming a vampire herself. The franchise's focus on the romantic struggles and the coming-of-age of a teenager appears obvious and resonates with its marketing as young adult fiction, despite being read well beyond the assigned age range of the field.[6] Yet supernatural elements, most prominently the Gothic figure of the vampire, seem to surpass clear-cut genre distinctions. Anne Morey explains that "Meyer is working with a combination of low-status genres – the vampire tale, the romance, the female coming-of-age-story" (2012: 2). Even so, *Twilight* intersects pop cultural references with canonic literary fiction, for instance, when using *Jane Eyre*'s Edward Rochester as inspiration for the vampire Edward (Valby 2009). Unsurprisingly, perhaps, the series also elicited interest in the subgenre that gives credit to its key ingredients: the paranormal ro-

---

5 *Twilight* has aptly been called a "Pop Culture Phenomenon" (Anatol 2011) and Melissa Click et al argue that "[d]espite its dismissal, the female-oriented *Twilight* franchise is comparable in profit and cultural impact to other well-respected media-franchises [...]" (2010: 6).

6 For further reference on *Twilight*'s readership beyond the market of young adults, refer to Leslie Paris: "Fifty Shades of Fandom: The Intergenerational Permeability of *Twilight* Fan Culture".

mance.[7] However, the vampire had already seized centerstage in the pop cultural realm before the publication of *Twilight*. Anne Rice's works or Charlaine Harris's *The Southern Vampire Mysteries* (2001–2013) exemplify vampires' potential to sell books and be adapted into film, with the former inspiring both the star-studded film *Interview with the Vampire* (1994) and an adaptation into an eponymous television series (2022), and HBO basing *True Blood* (2008–2014) on the latter. The vampire thus occurs in a variety of forms and genres and Nina Auerbach explains that "there is no such thing as 'The Vampire'; there are only vampires" (1997: 5).

Yet be they desirable or repulsive, burn in the sun or merely sparkle, vampires share a common feature: They do not age. Their non-aging turns them into a compelling point of reference for aging studies, as Sally Chivers explains in her discussion of aging and *Buffy, the Vampire Slayer*:

> Across traditions, vampires are typically immune to death from old age, maintain their age appearance from the time they were changed from humans into demons [...] As such, they offer an intriguing figure through which to separate a significant contemporary marker of old age – appearance – from a value that contemporary culture often ignores in older adults – experience. (2016: 89)

Here, Chivers remarks on vampires' capacity to present age via experience rather than physical markers, thereby allowing for a thorough discussion of age beyond physical change. As such, even though the vampire can be read as "old," they do not necessarily instill fears of dying as Auerbach contends: "Eternally alive, they embody not fear of death, but fear of life: Their power and their curse is their undying vitality" (1997: 5). The figure of the vampire is tied to ennui, with immortality showcasing the meaningfulness of the fleeting human lifespan – and in extension, granting value to aging.

---

7 For further reference on the sub-genre of paranormal romance see Joseph Crawford: *The Twilight of the Gothic?: Vampire Fiction and the Rise of the Paranormal Romance*: 6.

The vampire's non-aging gains further significance when read in the framework of their desirability. The attraction of the vampire was certainly not invented in Meyer's novels and is already suggested with Count Dracula entering women's bedrooms in Bram Stoker's constitutive work (1897). In Meyer's novels and in their adaptations, however, the desirability of the vampire lies at the core of the narrative as Bella and audience alike are invited to be humbled by the Cullens' beauty and grace. Here, age plays a significant role because youth and attractiveness are intricately linked throughout the series. Considering, for instance, Bella's reaction to Edward stating that he is over one hundred years old: "Well, maybe I shouldn't be dating such an old man. It's gross. I should be thoroughly repulsed" (Weitz 2010: 00:05:37). Her statement is followed by a lingering kiss and the sentiment's ironic nature is immediately revealed: Bella is far from being repulsed by Edward and their attraction is deliberately opposed to dating someone who would appear physically "old." Clearly, the vampire's non-aging intersects with his attractiveness, a connection that is crucial to all vampires depicted in the franchise. As Bella reminds her audience constantly of Edward's otherworldly appearance, to her, he is literally "a young god" (Meyer 2005: 299), his desirability cannot be separated from his apparent youth. The vampire, then, appears as a foil of glorified beauty set against Bella's aging human nature.

In the following, I further investigate the role of (non-)aging in the *Twilight* series and propose aging – not dying – as the true source of horror in both novels and their adaptations. This notion will be exemplified by two points of reference: A first part investigates Bella's unwillingness to grow older than Edward's seventeen years, and a second part discusses their daughter Renesmee's accelerated aging as a mirror of Bella's initial fears. Hereby, I aim at showing that *Twilight* introduces a heroine who is very much willing to die – but not to age. In effect, the series employs the vampires' arrested aging as an antidote to the horror of human aging and promotes internal maturation as a means to maintain both the stability of traditional social roles and the desirability of the seemingly young body.

"My wasted cheek": The Horror of Turning 18

Aging studies have underlined the ties between an aversion towards older age and a fear of death, with Heike Hartung and Rüdiger Kunow using the analogy of old age as a "'waiting room' in which people bide their time until they die" (2011: 18). Julia Velten further develops the metaphor and draws attention to the waiting room as a site of transition, thus signifying a "belonging nowhere" (2022: 24). Bella, who is witness to Edward's youthful perfection, already perceives herself in this waiting room at the age of seventeen. She remarks: "I'm dying already. Every second I get closer, older" (Hardwicke 2009: 01:46:48). Here, the vampire becomes an antidote to the fate of every human life and Bella's comment reveals a desire to avoid death and illness. Hereby, *Twilight* imagines an escape from the frailty of human life, as a remark by Anna Silver suggests: "As a breast cancer survivor, I found myself, as I read, wistfully longing for the possibility of my husband and I living forever in bodies that, unlike human bodies, do not age and sicken with disease" (2010: 137). Read in the context of human frailty, Bella's desire to become a vampire and to non-age illustrates a fear of death, however, her constant willingness to sacrifice herself points in another direction.

While Bella is deeply opposed to aging, her willingness to die is repeatedly emphasized in both novels and films. The desire to self-sacrifice is already established in the opening lines of the first film: "I'd never given much thought to how I would die, but dying in the place of someone I love seems like a good way to go" (Hardwicke 2009: 0:22). From the outset, Bella's path is connected to martyrdom, and she repeatedly establishes her firm belief that the most she can do is die for someone. For instance, she stabs herself to help Edward in his fight against Victoria (Meyer 2007: 488) and offers herself to a bloodthirsty vampire in an effort to save her mother (Meyer 2005: 375). Accordingly, Bonnie Mann explains that Meyer's novels "resurrec[t] the promise that a meaningful life comes *through* [emphasis in original] self-annihilation in the interest of others . . ." (2009: 144), and Bella's actions have been perceived to "embody Victorian values of female sacrifice for men" (Rocha 2014: 268). Fittingly, Brendan Shea links Bella's desire for immortality to her wish to care for her surroundings, "as her eventual death will prevent her from being there to protect and guide the people she loves" (2009: 80). Yet her clearly gendered willingness to die also suggests that Bella's desire to become a vampire and to non-age is not merely motivated by a fear of dying, but of aging. In the following, I want to draw attention to Bella's eighteenth birthday to illustrate this reading.

Turning eighteen is a rite of passage and bears legal significance: In the state of Washington, where *Twilight* is set, people reach adulthood at eighteen. While others might celebrate such an occasion, Bella is appalled by turning eighteen in the series' second installment, *New Moon* (2006). Her "dread" at reaching the age (Meyer 2006: 6) is, naturally, related to Edward's non-aging, his eternal seventeendom. In a conversation with his sister, Alice, this notion is exemplified:

> "What's the worst that could happen?" She meant it as a rhetorical question.
> "Getting older," I answered anyway, and my voice was not as steady as I wanted it to be.
> Beside me, Edward's smile tightened into a hard line.
> "Eighteen isn't very old," Alice said. "Don't women usually wait till they're twenty-nine to get upset over birthdays?"
> "It's older than Edward," I mumbled. (Meyer 2006: 9)

Bella's response to her imagining "the worst that could happen" establishes the underlying significance of aging in the series: The worst that could happen to Bella is "getting older". Alice's response is interesting in two regards, firstly, she situates Bella's fears against normative readings of age and, by suggesting that eighteen is still considered young, establishes that age operates within cultural frameworks. Secondly, she grants aging a specific gendered dimension as it is "women" who usually start worrying about their age before turning thirty. This notion is further underlined in the novel's filmic adaptation in which Emmet, Edward's brother, remarks at Bella's birthday party: "Dating an older woman, hot" (Weitz 2010: 00:13:23). As Susan Sontag has famously asserted with her "double standard of aging," aging cannot be separated from gender and impacts women harder than men (1972: 29). As Sontag emphasizes, this double standard is also closely entwined with female appearance and has a specifically aesthetic dimension (ibid: 31). Accordingly, Bella's desire to non-age hinges upon Edward's youth as an integral part of his attractiveness and she refuses to be immortalized as "a wrinkled little old lady" (Meyer 2006: 9). Clearly, youth is associated with beauty and power, while an aged appearance makes the imagined older Bella appear "little." Obviously, Bella wants to live with her partner forever, yet forever is appealing only in a body deemed young and, in effect, desirable.

This image of the visibly aged body as undesirable is prominently introduced in *New Moon*'s opening, when Bella dreams of herself as an aged woman next to Edward's unchanged image. In her dream, Bella looks at her grandmother, only to realize to her utter horror that she is encountering herself in a mirror:

> With a dizzying jolt, my dream abruptly became a nightmare. There was no Gran. That was *me* [emphasis in original]. Me in a mirror. Me – ancient, creased, and withered. Edward stood beside me, casting no reflection, excruciatingly lovely and forever seventeen. He pressed his icy, perfect lips against my wasted cheek. "Happy birthday," he whispered. (Meyer 2006: 6)

Bella's dream presents older age as a state of fearful decay and Ashley Benning explains that "now, Bella reveals her true concern: aging, and all that it entails" (2014: 91). In this regard, Benning fittingly speaks of Bella's "age phobia" and emphasizes that her "interpretation of aging includes illness, helplessness, senility, and becoming unattractive to Edward" (ibid: 91). In this scene, the difference between the non-aging vampire and decaying human could not be clearer: Whereas Edward's lips remain "perfect," Bella's cheek is "wasted." It is interesting to note that while Edward still appears as Bella's companion, he merely kisses her cheek in the novel, and in the film, he only brushes his lips to her hand (Weitz 2010: 00:03:04). Apparently, aged Bella does not receive a passionate kiss on the lips from the still-young vampire, rather, their relationship is established in almost asexual terms. Given that *Twilight* prominently features Bella's sexual desire for Edward, her threat of aging thus also equals a fear of sexual unattractiveness.

Hereby, the dream emphasizes that change is brought forth by age, so much so that Bella does not recognize herself: The aging self becomes someone else, someone unrecognizable. This foreignness relates to Margaret Morganroth Gullette's engagement with children reacting to "aged" versions of themselves at the Boston Science Museum. Gullette asserts that after encountering the virtually aged image shown on screen, "[t]he children were almost uniformly shaken" (2005: 4). The horror created by the distorting mirror appears reminiscent of Bella's despair upon realizing that she sees herself, rather than her grandmother. The feeling of not-self that Bella describes presents the aged self as abject, foreign and ultimately other.

Bella's dismay about her birthday, then, signifies her deep-seated horror of aging, a horror that is instilled by Edward's non-aging, and establishes the relational nature of age, namely that "[i]t always *takes two to age* [emphasis in original]" (Kunow 2011: 24). Bella's birthday turns her into an adult and further sets her apart from Edward whose seventeen years not only make him eternally adolescent but also relate to reading seventeen as a sexually desirable yet possibly still forbidden age.[8] Even though the vampire himself denies the reading of age as decay and constantly encourages Bella to stay human, he remains "perfect," the antithesis of Bella's fate of being "wasted" in older age. It thus appears that Bella is not merely afraid of dying, if dying young is an option – rather, she is afraid of dying *old*.

---

8   The age of seventeen has been featured at the intersection of adolescence and adulthood in a variety of forms in the pop cultural realm, for instance, in "17" Kings of Leon sing "Oh, she's only seventeen," indicating sexual desirability but also the forbidden nature of being a minor.

"Growing too fast": Renesmee's Accelerated Aging

In *Breaking Dawn* (2008) Bella finally becomes a vampire and one might expect her horror of aging to be over – yet, her fears take on a new form because her daughter, Renesmee, ages at an accelerated rate. In the following, I want to further investigate the role of Renesmee's accelerated aging and suggest that her aging is conceptualized in two distinct ways: in utero, it is read as uncontrollable growth and causes horror; once Renesmee is born, it is presented as maturing and creates a sense of wonder. Moreover, Bella's worry about her daughter's aging mirrors her previous fears and further strengthens the ties between female characters and a horror of growing older.

The fact that Renesmee grows at an accelerated speed is introduced in the moment that Bella realizes that she is pregnant. Only five days after her supposed menstruation, Bella begins to feel the fetus within her, a fact she deems "[i]mpossible" (Meyer 2008: 115). Yet, still in utero, the fetus grows rapidly, too rapidly for the human maternal body to accommodate and soon Bella's bones are broken from the inside (ibid: 294). The pregnancy alters the narrative's focus on the love triangle, a shift that is also expressed in form as Jacob becomes an interim narrator. His focus on Bella's withering body, her "mottled stomach" (ibid: 182), his assessment that "[y]ou'd think she was already dead" (ibid: 222) is mirrored in the film version's portrayal of Bella taking a bath with her skeletal body prominently displayed (Condon 2011: 01:13:39). These changes resonate with previous depictions of an unknown fetus as a source of horror, famously illustrated in *Rosemary's Baby* (1968). In Bella's case, the fetus appears horrifying primarily because of its incompatibility with the maternal body and its exceeding strength and growth. A conversation between Jakob and Edward, narrated by the former, underlines the link between the fetus' unknowable nature and its growth:

"The thing is ... growing. Swiftly. I can't be away from her now."
"What *is* [emphasis in original] it?"
"None of us have any idea. But it is stronger than she is. Already."

> I could suddenly see it then – see the swelling monster in my head, breaking her from the inside out. (Meyer 2008: 167–68)

To both shape shifter and vampire the horror associated with the unborn is prominently linked to its growth: It turns the fetus into "the thing" and a "swelling monster". This link between Renesmee and the monstrous is repeatedly underlined, for instance by the werewolves who deem the fetus "[u]nnatural. Monstrous" (Meyer 2008: 183) and plan on killing the half-vampire as they "don't know what kind of creature the Cullens have bred, but [they] know that it is strong and fast-growing" (ibid: 184). Again, the fetus' accelerated maturation serves as the basis for skepticism and horror. As a half-vampire, Renesmee's nature appears utterly unknown, yet it is her growth that immediately identifies her as dangerous.

Once Renesmee is born, the horror her surroundings feel is soon replaced by a sense of wonder. Now, references to the monstrous, as suggested by her nickname "Nessie," appear humoristic rather than chilling. At the same time, her developments are no longer framed as uncontrolled growth, rather she is presented as growing into maturity (ibid: 549). Lisa Nevárez accordingly understands her as "balancing between the innocent child and the startingly mature one" (2013: 113) and explains that Renesmee "looks like a child and can do childish things but who contains a very adult nature" (2013: 117). Even though the Cullens are still continuously surprised by her development, her growth – or maturation, as it is now called – no longer instills a sense of threat. Compared to his previous assessment of the fetus as "the thing ... growing," Edward now describes Renesmee's development as a source of wonder: "She's intelligent, shockingly so, and progressing at an immense pace. Though she doesn't speak – yet – she communicates quite effectively" (Meyer 2008: 397). While previously, Renesmee's aging was predominantly linked to "growth" – as a physical characteristic –, it is now framed in the terms of "progress" and relates to her intelligence. Renesmee thus becomes, as Benning notes, "almost a peer to her aunts and uncles" (2014: 93) and her chronological age of a few months is surpassed by her maturity. While the fetus' "growth" presented cause for concern in relation to Bella's body,

Renesmee's "progress" presents a threat to herself. It is her accelerated aging, and the entailed possibility of her premature demise, that triggers the family's worry and connects to Bella's already established "age phobia" (ibid: 91).

As Bella worries about her daughter's lifespan, she also revisits her deep-seated fears of aging and frames older age as the ultimate form of human decay. Accordingly, she understands her daughter's accelerated age process in terms of fixed phases:

> By Carlisle's calculations, the growth of her body was gradually slowing; her mind continued to race on ahead. Even if the rate of decrease held steady, she'd still be an adult in no more than four years. Four years. And an old woman by fifteen.
> Just fifteen years of life. (Meyer 2008: 490)

Again, a teenager's life is assessed with reference to aging, and again, becoming "an old woman" appears as a nightmarish scenario. While Bella's fear of aging prominently relied on Edward as a foil of eternal youth, Renesmee's aging is opposed to what her mother expects and to what can be assumed to be "normal" aging. As such, Bella's shock about being "an old woman by fifteen" relies on cultural framings of adolescence contrasting older age. These frames gain further significance against the backdrop of Bella's immortality: Read in this context, Renesmee's aging appears as a distorted mirror of her mother's previous fears. Even though her accelerated aging might present her as utterly different from the rest of her family, it still functions as a metaphor for the progressing human lifespan. Her aging, then, serves as the ultimate reminder of human frailty and presents Renesmee not only as different, but also as hyper-human. With her daughter, Bella's nightmare of turning into her grandmother has returned: She imagines her daughter old and – as we may conclude from her previous reading of her own aged body – "wasted."

Despite her immortality, undeniable beauty and eternal youth, aging thus again presents the sole opponent in Bella's life. As she explains in voice-over: "It seemed like we only had one enemy left: Time. Renesmee was growing too fast" (Condon 2012: 29:34). Aging is framed as the "enemy" that stands in the way of the young family's happiness, and the importance granted to time is tied to the changes it instills in Renesmee, who grows "too" fast. Here, Renesmee's aging is pathologized, a notion also prominently suggested by Carlisle's studies of her development. It is unsurprising that the changes brought by the "enemy time" are unsettling to Bella who comments after not seeing Renesmee for a night: "Abruptly, something close to panic had my body freezing up. What would she look like today?" (Meyer 2008: 450). Her accelerated aging turns Renesmee into an Other: Reminiscent of her reaction to her aged image in the mirror, Bella is afraid of what her daughter's aged version might look like. While Renesmee's maturity is thus appreciated, her aging is a source for "panic" and Bella explains: "The thought of Renesmee's speeding life had me stressed out again in an instant" (ibid: 451). Similarly, watching an animated growth-spurt, the film's audience is invited to follow Bella's line of thought and to wonder just how long the child might live (Condon 2012: 29:34). Following Xavier Aldana Reyes's understanding that "[h]orror takes its name, in other words, from the effects that it seeks to elicit in its readers" (2016: 7), the horror presented here is that of aging.

In conclusion, Renesmee's aging is presented along different frames of meaning-making: it instills both threat and fear, but contrastingly, when read as maturation, her aging is also commendable and marks her as non-threatening. In fact, Renesmee's aging, or her becoming mature, is vital to the Cullens' defense against the Volturi and to their attempt to prove that she is not an immortal (and full-vampire) child (Meyer 2008: 549). In this instance, her aging – and the ties to humanity it signifies – is key to her survival. In the case of Renesmee, aging moves beyond presenting the horror it did to her mother, even though this reading is still apparent. More specifically, her not behaving childlike, and thus not "acting her age," makes it acceptable that she will eventually stop aging.

Conclusion: The Vampire as an Antidote to Horror

What, then, can be gleaned about aging as horror in *Twilight Saga*? As Bella's fear of aging suggests, signs of older age create a sense of horror in the young heroine who deems herself "wasted" next to Edward's perfection – and eternal youth. At first glance, Renesmee's accelerated aging appears as a mirror of these fears given that Bella's aging is replaced by fear for her daughter's life.

Yet Renesmee also illustrates that maturation creates a sense of wonder rather than horror and thereby exemplifies a correct timeframe to stop aging: A timeframe that neither includes childhood nor older age. In fact, while older age is linked to decay, childlike behavior is repeatedly dismissed as undesirable, considering, for instance, Edward calling Jakob "a pup" when annoyed with him (Meyer 2007: 303). Here, the divergence between what can be understood as experienced age and chronological age comes to the fore, an opposition that Benning addresses by speaking of "physically mature but emotionally stunted wolves, or the intellectually mature but physically stunted vampires" (2014: 92). In fact, Bella only perceives Jakob as "plenty mature" once she allows her romantic feelings for him (Meyer 2007: 520). Youth, when read as immaturity, remains undesirable and possibly even dangerous, as is showcased in the threat posed by immortal children. Maturation, in contrast, is presented as highly commendable, as suggested by the protagonist Bella who was "born thirty-five years old" (Meyer 2005: 91), is emotionally mature and in effect takes care of both of her parents.[9] If Bella was to be considered childish, as, for instance, the clichéd teenager Jessica, she would neither be a fitting mate for Edward nor appear mature enough for immortality.

Twilight suggests, then, that the right time to become a vampire and to escape the horrors of aging occurs at the intersection of emotional maturation and youthful attractiveness and sexual desirability. While their stunted aging might transgress notions of age-appropriateness, the societal functions the Cullens perform clearly adhere to age tropes: They finish high school repeatedly, they are all matched in heterosexual

---

9   For further reference on Bella's role as a caregiver see Silver: 124.

relationships and not only perform the roles of siblings and parents, rather, they understand their ties as familial. Fittingly, Benning explains that they "have created a system to mimic that of a mortal family" (2014: 95). In conclusion, they are stunted at the time they can best contribute to their community, be it economically – they are constantly buying cars and clothes – or socially, with Carlisle being a doctor. The horror that *Twilight* elicits of older age thereby resonates with readings typically associated with "senior citizens": Aside from unattractiveness, it alludes to not contributing to society. Thus, *Twilight*'s vampires oppose the horror of aging in two distinct regards: They not only promise eternal beauty, but on a societal level, they counter fears of "aging populations" and what has been called "a silver tsunami" (Rotman 2019).

In the series' end, the horror of aging ceases to have a hold on Bella as she fully grasps that her daughter will stop aging, too. It is only then that *Breaking Dawn* concludes with a chapter titled "The Happily Ever After" and leaves the couple in their cottage in the woods. In German, fairytales do not end on "happily ever after," they conclude with: "Und wenn sie nicht gestorben sind, dann leben sie noch heute," which translates into "and if they have not died yet, they are still alive today." While this fairytale ending interweaves the happy end with the possibility of death, *Twilight* allows for the ultimate "Happily Ever After": Bella and Edward do not have to die – even better – they do not have to age.

Author Bio

Ruth Gehrmann is a postdoctoral researcher in the CRC "Studies in Human Categorization" at Johannes Gutenberg-University Mainz, Germany where she works on a project on Aging Studies. She holds a PhD in American Studies and is specifically interested in popular culture and the medical humanities.

Works Cited

Anatol, Giselle Liza (2011): "Introduction." In: Giselle Liza Anatol (ed.), Bringing Light to Twilight: Perspectives on a Pop Culture Phenomenon, New York: Palgrave Macmillan, pp. 1–11.
Auerbach, Nina (1997): Our Vampires, Ourselves. Chicago: University of Chicago Press.
Benning, Ashley (2014): "'How Old Are You?' Representations of Age in the Saga." In: Maggie Parke/Natalie Wilson (eds.), Theorizing Twilight: Critical Essays on What's at Stake in a Post-Vampire World, Jefferson: McFarland, pp. 87–101.
Chivers, Sally (2016): "'Vampires Don't Age, But Actors Sure Do.' The Cult of Youth and the Paradox of Aging in Buffy the Vampire Slayer." In: Maricel Oró-Piqueras/Anita Wohlmann (eds.), Serializing Age, Aging Studies 7, pp. 89–107.
Click, Melissa A./Jennifer Stevens Aubrey/Elizabeth Behm-Morawitz (2010): "Introduction." In: Melissa A. Click/Jennifer Stevens Aubrey/Elizabeth Behm-Morawitz (eds.), Bitten by Twilight, New York: Peter Lang, pp. 1–17.
Condon, Bill, dir. (2011): Breaking Dawn, Part 1.
Condon, Bill, dir. (2012): Breaking Dawn, Part 2.
Crawford, Joseph (2014): The Twilight of the Gothic?: Vampire Fiction and the Rise of the Paranormal Romance. Cardiff: University of Wales Press.
Gullette, Margaret Morganroth (2005): Aged by Culture. Chicago: University Press.
Hardwicke, Catherine, dir. (2009): Twilight.
Hartung, Heike, and Rüdiger Kunow (2011): "Introduction: Age Studies." Amerikastudien/American Studies 56/1, pp. 15–22.
Kings of Leon, "17", January 1, 2017 (https://www.youtube.com/watch?v=5Y9kJzJ8Emk)
Kunow, Rüdiger (2011): "Chronologically Gifted? 'Old Age' in American Culture." Amerikastudien/American Studies 56/1, pp. 23–44.
Mann, Bonnie (2009): "Vampire Love: The Second Sex Negotiates the Twenty-First Century." In: Rebecca Housel/J. Jeremy Wisnewski

(eds.), Twilight and Philosophy: Vampires, Vegetarians, and the Pursuit of Immortality, Hoboken: John Wiley & Sons, pp. 131–45.
Meyer, Stephenie (2005): Twilight. London: atom.
Meyer, Stephenie (2006): New Moon. London: atom.
Meyer, Stephenie (2007): Eclipse. London: atom.
Meyer, Stephenie (2008): Breaking Dawn. London: atom.
Morey, Anne (2012): "Introduction." In: Anne Morey (ed.), Genre, Reception, and Adaptation in the "Twilight" Series, London: Routledge, pp. 1–14.
Nevárez, Lisa (2013): "Renesmee as (R)omantic Child: A Glimpse into Bella and Edward's Fairy Tale Cottage." In: Claudia Bucciferro (ed.), The Twilight Saga: Exploring the Global Phenomenon, Lanham: Scarecrow Press, pp. 107–21.
Paris, Leslie (2016): "Fifty Shades of Fandom: The Intergenerational Permeability of Twilight Fan Culture." Feminist Media Studies 16/4, pp. 678–92.
Reyes, Xavier Aldana (2016): "Introduction: What, Why and When Is Horror Fiction." In: Xavier Aldana Reyes (ed.), Horror: A Literary History, London: British Library Publishing, pp. 7–17.
Rocha, Lauren (2014): "Wife, Mother, Vampire: The Female Role in the Twilight Series." Journal of International Women's Studies 15/2, pp. 286–98.
Rotman, David (2019): "Why You Shouldn't Fear the Gray Tsunami." MIT Technology Review. August 21, 2019. https://www.technologyreview.com/2019/08/21/133311/why-you-shouldnt-fear-the-gray-tsunami/.
Shea, Brendan (2009): "To Bite or Not to Bite: Twilight, Immortality, and the Meaning of Life." In: Rebecca Housel/J. Jeremy Wisnewski, Twilight and Philosophy: Vampires, Vegetarians, and the Pursuit of Immortality, Hoboken: John Wiley and Sons, pp. 79–93.
Silver, Anna (2010): "Twilight Is Not Good for Maidens: Gender, Sexuality, and the Family in Stephenie Meyer's Twilight Series." Studies in the Novel 42/1–2, pp. 121–39.
Sontag, Susan (1972): "The Double Standard of Aging." The Saturday Review, pp. 29–38.

spirt_mage_234. 2009. "Why Twilight is NOT Gothic Literature." Livejournal. May 18, 2009. https://twilight-sucks.livejournal.com/757050.html.

Valby, Karen (2009): "Stephenie Meyer: 12 of My 'Twilight' Inspirations." EW.Com. September 28, 2009 (https://ew.com/gallery/stephenie-meyer-12-my-twilight-inspirations/)

Velten, Julia (2022): Extraordinary Forms of Aging. Bielefeld: transcript.

Weitz, Chris, dir. (2010): New Moon.

Claudia: The Forever Child and Vampire Killer in Anne Rice's *Interview with the Vampire*

Kimberly Smith[1]

> "The Ruthless Pursuit of Blood with all of a Child's Demanding" (Rice 1997: 96)

The vampire, the quintessential gothic character, never ages; he is paradoxically "the living dead." The allure of the vampiric figure is that he defeats aging and death, a trait most desired by humans. He is playing with evil by attempting to overthrow God's or the universe's natural order. Barbara Fray Waxman discusses how vampires simultaneously fascinate and challenge us because, "They are ... vehicles to explore the *Tabula Rasa* condition of twentieth-century human existence, as well as the quest for truths, moral rules, and a purposeful existence" (Waxman 1992: 82). The modern vampire's popularity has become the symbol of the fears and anxieties of modern-day culture and society.

In the modern age, representations of the vampire have not been old and fearful but young, beautiful, sexy, and dangerous. Youthful depictions of vampires began in earnest with the novels written by Anne Rice, who created a world of male vampires who were young, adventurous, and dangerously attractive. Rice made it a rule that vampires only "turned" those who were youthfully beautiful while introducing this

---

1 Elizabeth City State University.

risqué but alarmingly alluring depiction of the vampire. Rice revolutionized the vampire genre by giving the vampire a voice and focusing more on him than the vampire victims. Young, sexy, and alluring vampires have been depicted in literature, such as Sheridan Le Fanu's *Carmilla* (1872). However, until Anne Rice reinvented the genre by focusing on his youth, little attention was paid to the vampire's age. Pop culture immediately gravitated to this new semblance of that fabled fictional character.

The vampire has fascinated us for ages because of our conflicting feelings towards death. Whether one believes in the hereafter or not, no one has taken that final sojourn of life and returned to present a bird's eye view. In Hamlet's famous "To Be or Not to Be" speech, he says,

> But that the dread of something after death
> The undiscovere'd country, from whose bourn
> No traveller returns, puzzles the will... (William Shakespeare 1603:1)

Undoubtedly, this innate fear of many people cannot be more profoundly expressed than through the words of Shakespeare. Because of this fear, one can easily understand how engaging the promise of eternal life is to humanity. Of all the horror monsters, the one that has mesmerized society the most is the vampire. Why? To society, the vampire defies death and age, allowing people to live within their familiar reality. The vampire that intrigues people the most is aristocratic, young, or youngish, so much so that he can assimilate within human society almost always undistinguishable and undisturbed. No one wants eternity as an old elderly person stuck perpetually in the deficits of the aging body. Instead, people desire everlasting youth enshrined forever. The vampire's life approximates earthly human life while enjoying eternity.

Because of this youthful depiction, Rice's work has known unrivaled popularity. Unfortunately, the female vampire does not share the stage equally with the males in Rice's male-dominated vampire universe. However, within Anne Rice's world, there are female vampires, and of these, the most tragically infamous is Claudia, who appears in the first novel of the Vampire Chronicles, *Interview with The Vampire*.[2] The novel centers on Louis de Pointe du Lac, who is being interviewed about his life. He recounts his relationships with Lestat de Lioncourt, who "turned" him into a vampire, woefully describing his dual status in Claudia's life as father/lover. Claudia, who is "turned" into a vampire at five, was created from Rice's grief for her daughter, Michelle, who died from leukemia [at age 5]. (Jowett, 2). Grieving beyond measure, Rice developed a fictional character of a child who would not die.

With Claudia's introduction to the vampire world came critical analysis concerning aging and its effect on the child vampire through issues such as sexuality, adulthood, innocence, and the killer instinct – complex elements that simultaneously complement and threaten her existence. The vampire child ages mentally yet is stymied by a child's body. How does society process this child-like being with a woman's appetite yet with a killer's mind? Childhood is a temporary but essential stage of life that helps us learn skills and mental processes that enable us to move successfully into adulthood. The dichotomy of the vampire child is that it is stuck in this temporary state forever, clashing mentally with its physical body – robbed eternally of the opportunity to blossom in the natural state of childhood. Not only is the problem that others see her as a child, but her mental maturity is at stake as well. Mentally, she vacillates between a child's tantrums and an adult's thoughts and wants. This chapter looks at the complexity of Claudia as a literary vampire character and the problems that inevitably arise from dealing with her conflicting physical and mental states as she ages mentally yet remains physically stagnant, especially her depiction in film and television, where the visual is constant.

By studying Claudia's images in the novel, film, and AMC television series, one can see the difficulty in addressing the vampire child within

---

2 When *Interview with the Vampire* was published in 1976, there were still very few female vampires in literature. One of the most important and earliest was *Carmilla* (1872) by Sheridan Le Fanu. Its main importance is that a female vampire is at the center, but there is also a child victim.

the traditional idea of horror and aging – inclusively, the subject of sexuality as it emerges in her relationship with Louis. Focusing on Claudia's two most defining aspects – aging and sexuality – I will analyze and critique her depiction as she evolves in the legendary world of vampire horror. Therefore, this chapter critiques Claudia as she is depicted from the five-year-old in the novel to the ten-year-old in the film and ultimately to the fourteen-year-old in the AMC series, respectively. In discussing her evolution, she will be analyzed first as she develops mentally as a mature woman yet absent of any physical statuette. Secondly, this analysis of Claudia will examine her as a ten-year-old, with particular reference to the impact of the visual medium of film as it reflects on the contrasting elements of her thwarted life as a child vampire – characterized by sexual/mental mutability versus childlike physical inertia. Lastly, Claudia will be assessed at fourteen as the teenage/biracial vampire represented in a continual episodic television series, with no end game – compelling the use of melodramatic tropes, i.e., teenage rebellion, to attract a loyal viewing audience. These depictions of Claudia have positioned her at a different age for the crucially defining and the fatal point in her life – the "turning" – while justifying her creation as one of the most tragically portrayed legends in vampire horror fiction.

Within the Gothic genre, aging is depicted as premature or a supernatural element, and elderly people are seen within the mystic world as victims. The child vampire can be just as disarming as an elderly mask or person because of "The monstrous disjunction of a young body with an old consciousness, or a 'child usurping adult desires, prerogatives, or power... (McDevitt 2020: 220). The child has always been one of the most unsettling aspects of Gothic fiction because innocence masks evil within this childlike visual image.

The horror child is seemingly an aberration of nature, but the vampire child is different – she is "something else" because she has an adult mind; she can use her child's innocence to lure her victims. She is more calculating in her evil acts. As she develops mentally, but not physically, she plots, manipulates, and connives; therefore, maximizing the use of her arrested childhood looks to take advantage of the unsuspected.

Furthermore, youth is highly prized within society, especially by women. However, what happens if a woman is too young or looks too young? This, of course, is the case with the vampire child, aging mentally but not physically. Scholars Horner and Zslick stated that the "Othering' of the self is partly due to the recognition of inevitable physical change and decay in one's own body and the sense of split subjectivity it can produce and partly to the acceptance of social attitudes which see the old as irrelevant and as an (increasingly heavy) economic burden" (Horner and Zsolick 2016: 184–185). Although the vampire child does not need to fear aging, there is the fear of not having the inevitable change in one's body. Just as the elderly are seen as irrelevant, so is the vampire child. Children can be seen as a nuisance and a problem for working parents; often, they are a source of conflict within a family and must be watched to avoid danger, etc. For most of childhood, children are little people who are dependent upon their elders; they have very little autonomy over what goes on in their environment. This is the crux of the vampire child who will be all the above for eternity. Claudia's physical body will always be an obstacle to becoming a genuine vampire with all the accouterments, such as complete agency.

Undeniably, the core of the vampire construct since Dracula has been sexuality. But when American films seized the vampire, they focused heavily on making the vampire an aristocratic, alluring, and captivating man. The monster aspect was sometimes de-emphasized to entice the audience to connect to the vampire. Consequently, the portrayer of a vampire since Bela Lugosi has usually been a handsome, supernatural sex symbol.

Additionally, the theme of vampire sexuality continues in the evolution of Claudia. Intrinsically linked to the depiction of Claudia as the child vampire is always the undercurrent of sexuality, which inherently leads to apprehensions about child exploitation. How do you portray adult sexuality within the body of a child? As society has become more aware of the sexual trafficking of children and teenagers, representing the vampire child becomes more problematic. Additionally, society does not want to acknowledge any sexuality with children. Children are innocent, so they should not be spoiled or tainted by sexuality. Because the child vampire is both prey and predator, dealing with her sexuality is awkwardly challenging.

Interview with the Vampire (novel, 1976)

From Claudia's first appearance in the novel, one senses the combined elements of tragedy and victimization. Claudia is brought into the novel by Louis, who attacks her as an innocent five-year-old child crying over her dead mother. Later, Lestat finds a sick Claudia, which, in a fit of impulse, leads him to give her the dark gift of immortality. The theft of a child's innocence is startling, even in a vampire novel. This is the beginning of Claudia losing her childhood. A stolen childhood can never be retrieved; the basis for forming the child into adulthood has been lost forever. Claudia has no foundation to build upon because she has been turned into the "monster" at an unknowing age. As Lestat makes a self-serving choice, the dye is cast, and this child prey suddenly becomes a child predator.

The reader agonizes as one envisions Claudia's transformation from a small child to an adult woman still within her diminutive frame. Claudia strives futilely to become the woman she desires to be. The ultimate goal of the child is to become an adult. For the child, adulthood is seen as independence to make her own life choices. Unfortunately, because of the conflict between her mental state and her physical being, Claudia can never achieve true independence. On the contrary, the reader is also amazed at how she uses her childish look to lure unknowing victims to their deaths at her hands. Because no matter how frustrated she is because of her static place, she relies on her instincts to survive, as only vampires can – to find and kill her prey, humans.

Initially, the reader visualizes Claudia as a flesh and blood child with her eyes looking imploringly to Louis for help. Louis states, "...I had bent down and driven hard onto her small soft neck and, hearing her tiny cry, whispered even as I felt the hot blood on my lips, 'It's only for a moment, and there will be no more pain'" (Rice 1997: 73). This passage illustrates the vulnerability of the child to a predator. Even though Louis is sympathetic, his very nature as a vampire and a predator takes precedence over any latent humanistic apprehensions. Because of her age and size, Claudia is prey via a multitude of dimensions.[3]

After Lestat "turns" Claudia by having her drink his blood, she says in her little girl's voice, "I want some more..." (Rice 1997: 93). From this moment, she is now the vampire child. Here, the dichotomy between the vampire and the child takes hold because Claudia has rapidly developed a "thirst for blood." As a child, Claudia characteristically wants more of something that she likes. However, the novelty is that the "something" is blood.

She assumes the role of a vampire immediately. Louis tells the interviewer, "... I couldn't comprehend her; for little child she was, but also fierce killer now capable of the ruthless pursuit of blood with all a child's demanding" (Rice 1997: 96). These words convey the irony of the vampire child. Although she still has childish instincts, they are now infused with the evil intent of the vampire to kill. In fact, being a child makes her associate with evil in a more basic way. Children are by nature selfish, do not have a fully developed consciousness, and do not see any other view other than their own. Since becoming a vampire so young, she does not develop human qualities. Louis, who understands what it means to be human, cannot comprehend how quickly Claudia has developed a taste for this morbid life. Unlike Louis, Claudia is not burdened with the human conflicts of right and wrong.

---

3   The novel *Carmilla* also has a child victim, but her attack is depicted as a dreamlike sequence while she sleeps. The main character, Laura, remembers when she was six years old that a woman came and bit her, but she feels it was a dream. Towards the end of the novel, she has another dreamy episode where she is bitten on her chest. In the 19th century, La Fanu was investigating the idea of a child victim and an adult predator. Although not bitten in a dream, Claudia is similar to Laura because her second attack is in bed. There is a clear similarity between Laura and Claudia because the sexual vampire construct frames both victims.

Although not planned, Louis, Lestat, and now Claudia form an unconventional vampire family.[4] This family stability is endangered when Claudia learns the truth about her creation. She takes her vengeance out on the man she considers the culprit, Lestat, the robber of her mortal self. Nevertheless, this structure also becomes problematized as Claudia grows up mentally and realizes that she will never be independent of her "fathers". Anne Rice says, "The child vampire Claudia was physically inspired by Michelle, but she ultimately became something else – a woman trapped in a child's body, robbed of power, never knowing what it's like to really be a woman and make love. She became a metaphor for a raging mind trapped in a powerless body...." (Qtd in Jowett 2002: 59). Claudia cannot exist as she is, and she knows it. She will not have immortality because the dichotomy between her mental maturity and her child body cannot co-exist forever.

Another problematic area of Claudia's identity that will become more of an issue once she is depicted in the film is her sexuality. Sexuality has been the primary focus of the vampire model in film since Bela Lugosi's version of *Dracula* in 1931. When Louis first sees her, he says, "But the question pounded in me: Am I damned? If so, why do I feel such pity for her, for her gaunt face? Why do I wish to touch her tiny, soft arms, hold her now on my knee as I am doing, feel her bend her head to my chest as I gently touch the satin hair" (Rice 1997: 73)? This passage vacillates between Louie feeling pity for the child, wanting to attack her, and having a latent sexual interest.

---

4   The construct of a family created out of victimization relates to the Netflix movie *May December* (2023). Gracie Atherton-Yoo seduces a 12-year-old, Joe Yoo, and becomes pregnant. Years later, they marry when Joe becomes an adult. This is an unconventional family with sexually inappropriate overtones. Even though Claudia is in a vampire family, she is in the same position as Joe in many ways. She was victimized at a young age when consent was not possible. She creates a family with the men who are, in one way, her predators, and eventually, like Joe, she will become involved romantically with one of them, Louis. How can Claudia or Joe process the role of a victim who creates a relationship with his/her predator?

Although she is still in the body of a five-year-old, as Claudia matures mentally, Louis envisions her as the woman she becomes as they eventually become lovers. When reading the novel, it is less awkward to view Claudia as a maturing vampire than it is in a screen adaptation. As one reads the work, one hears Claudia's voice as she matures (without the visual of the face) so the reader can access the imagination without the intrusion of the physical as is shown in the film. The image of the five-year-old is kept at bay. As stated earlier, when the novel was written, the sexualization of minors within pop culture was not an issue that was critiqued. As time has progressed and cultural changes have evolved, filmmakers and television producers have been confronted with this undeniably relevant yet highly controversial aspect. Claudia cannot ever grow up – "suspended" forever in childhood." Even though she develops mentally, she can never assume her adult role. Not assuming her adult role will eclipse Claudia's life until her untimely death. Claudia can never truly know what she wants. Her suspension in childhood challenges her love for Loue. She will never have the choice to see if she wants someone else or if her choice is truly to be with Louis.

Interview With the Vampire (1994)

In 1994, Neil Jordan was pegged to direct a film version of the widely popular novel, casting Tom Cruise as Lestat, Brad Pitt as Louis, and Kirsten Dunst as Claudia. For the character of Claudia, Jordan aged her to 10, and Dunst was 12 when she played the part. In the DVD commentary, Neil Jordan said he needed to ensure he had a true actress for the role. (*Interview with the Vampire film*) However, even the 12-year-old Dunst had problems with the latent sexuality of the part. Vicki Fenn states, "Dunst clearly had issues with being required to act like a woman when she herself was no such thing," (Fenn 2021:64).

Of course, confronted with these sensitive and possibly volatile possibilities, the film industry has increasingly sought a means to depict the issue of sexuality without seemingly promoting child exploitation. As in the novel and "In the film, the strongest erotic bonding is between Louis and Claudia." (Pintillie 2015:129). The latent sexuality appears early in the film when Claudia is "turned" by Lestat. Although Claudia is depicted as an object in both the book and the movie, visual imagery, of course, takes precedence in the movie. Her transition in the film occurs when Lestat brings Louis to their place and sees Claudia sleeping in the bed. Thinking he killed her, Louis is stunned to see her there. Immediately, Lestat talks about how wonderful she looks and what it would be like to "take" her. Lestat presents Claudia to Louis as a delectable food. The whole setup reeks of an undercurrent of sexuality. Lestat takes the bull by the horns when Louis refuses to relieve her of her suffering and "turns" her into a vampire. Watching the vulnerable child turn into a monster is where the absolute horror of the movie begins.

In time, Louis and Claudia become lovers in the book and movie, i.e., Dunst's kissing scene with Brad Pitt. Scholar Violet Fenn states, "...It is the very presence of Claudia that gives *Interview* its uneasy tone. In modern culture, vampires are generally depicted as being inherently sexual. The juxtaposition of an immortal mind in a prepubescent body is an uncomfortable one. But regardless of ethics, the fact remains that Claudia, as a character, *is* an adult woman who simply has an outward appearance of a child" (Fenn 202:64). It is understood that she is mentally an adult by the time Claudia and Louis become lovers.[5] But as depicted in the film, when Lestat "turns" her, there is a sexualization of Claudia, the child. Of course, within the visual development of the love story between Louis and Claudia and the intimate sexuality, the audience is cinematically directed to focus on her implied mature adult status in lieu of Claudia's visual childlike persona.[6]

---

5   The contradictory relationship that is seen with Claudia and Louis can also be seen with Carmilla and Laura in *Carmilla*. When Laura is bitten the first time she does not know who did it or even if it happened because she thinks it was a dream, but when Carmilla, the vampire predator, comes to her family in the body of a woman, she and Laura develop an uneasy yet close relationship.

6   This connects strongly to the movie *May December* because Claudia is now in a relationship with her predator, just as Joe was in a relationship with Grace, his predator. He was sexualized as a child, just as Claudia is sexualized. Joe

The other central theme of the film is the construction of a child killer. One scene that emphasizes the dichotomy of her internal growth as a killer and her child-like visage and body occurs when she is having her dress made by her dressmaker. The dressmaker accidentally cuts her finger, and Claudia is immediately drawn to the blood. When the scene shifts back to her, the dressmaker is dead, and Claudia has a coyly innocent look that could easily rival Shirley Temple.

Claudia is a killer in the mold of Lestat, not Louis. Since her transformation as a vampire occurs as a child, she quickly masters her required "killing skills," disdainfully rejecting all remorse for her actions. Her child's temperament, combined with her deadly instinct, is fascinating to watch. Claudia's physical embodiment of the white, cute, blonde-curled little girl belies the fact that these physical traits walk in tandem with the internal blood-sucking characteristics of a vampire. Claudia's curly blonde hair conjures up a dark image of the Shirley Temple look. It is a crucial portrait because it aids in subverting the true Claudia: a bona fide vampire killer. Aided and abetted by this visual image of whiteness, society is waylaid when confronted with the real Claudia. A black child of the same age and circumstances would not be seen this innocently. Claudia's evilness is wrapped in whiteness.

As Claudia matures, she realizes what she will never be. This is first seen during a nighttime outing. Claudia spots a naked Creole young woman by her bedroom window. For the first time, there is a recognition of the difference between her and an adult-looking woman. Lestat notices that Claudia is studying the woman and asks her:

"Do you want her?"
Claudia states, "No, I want to be her. Can I, Louis, be her someday?"
(*Interview With the Vampire*, film)

As mutual culprits, Louis and Lestat bear responsibility for Claudia's fragmented and double identity and are fully aware that she will never

---

was trapped once Grace was pregnant with his child, and Claudia was trapped when she was turned into a vampire.

realize her dream. Although this scene in the film is not in the book, it is critical to understanding Claudia's conflicting situations.[7] The film better illustrates her eternal conflict and frustration: the Creole woman represents what Claudia can never be – a physically mature woman. Conforming to her body size, Lestat continues to dress her as a little girl or a China doll. She is never even allowed to look the part of her physical maturity. Rebelling against Lestat's form of subjugation, seething with rage, Claudia angrily denounces Lestat for his insistence on keeping her as the little girl.[8] Unabated, Lestat continually gives her dolls because that is what she is – the "eternal doll.' (Jordan DVD Commentary). She will never experience the human existence of growing up or the vampire coming of age.

One of the critical scenes in the film occurs when Claudia first confronts Lestat. Screaming at him, she furiously takes all the dolls off her bed to reveal the dead Creole woman; Claudia, who has been drawing pictures of the woman, craves to be her. In many ways, Claudia likens the woman's decaying corpse in her bed to her dream of becoming an adult woman. However, her dream has become decayed, twisted, and grotesque, just like the Creole woman's body. It is a dream not just deferred but forever denied. In her fury over the realization of her state, she "cuts her childish curls off, but her hair grows back in an instant as the film demonstrates to the audience that Claudia can never change from

---

7   This recognition scene with Claudia is similar to the one in the movie *May December*. Joe is sitting on the roof of his house and having a talk with his son, Charlie, before he goes to college. Charlie offers his father a joint and is surprised that he has never smoked one. At that moment, Joe realizes what he has lost, accepting he will never return to his adolescence. He is forever in between childhood and adulthood. He realizes for the first time how Grace's manipulations irrevocably changed his life, just as Claudia realizes what she will never be and who is responsible.

8   Claudia rages at Lestat for turning her into a vampire and is hurt to realize Louis was a part of her "turning." Claudia confronts both men, and Joe confronts Grace in *May December*. Grace deflects the criticism, blaming him for the situation. She, in fact, says that Joe seduced her. Unlike Lestat, who owns what he did, Grace refuses to take responsibility.

the physical shape she had when Lestat turned her into a vampire" (Reep, etc. !996:130). From the point that she becomes a vampire, Claudia's life tragically worsens.

As Louis and Claudia sit in the New Orleans night air, people watching, they see an old woman. Believing he is casting away any of Claudia's anxiety about aging, Louis tells her that she will never grow old. Refutably, she responds that she will never grow up. (*Interview with the Vampire film*) Claudia's issues with being unable to grow up seem antithetical to understanding the vampire, age, and aging in society. When discussing the Twilight books, one of the significant issues for "... feminist readers, [is] Bella Swan's reasons for wishing to be transformed into a vampire herself include not only the desire to be with her vampire hero, Edward, forever but also a terrible fear of aging: her worst nightmare..." (Horner and Zlosnik 2016:188). When Louis directs Claudia's attention to the old woman, he sees the old woman in the mode of the Gothic and society as irrelevant. He believes that Claudia should revel in always being young and should be relieved that she will not have the fate of being seen as a burden or as serviceably futile in society. Taking no pleasure or satisfaction from Louis's promise of eternal youth, Claudia feels that as the woman in the child's body, she is just as useless as the old woman.

Eventually, Louis and Claudia move to Paris, which, of course, is where complicated issues develop because "the film, in using an eleven-year-old actress instead of a five-year-old, strengthens the pedophilia implications that appear in the novel and, at the same time, creates the image of a tragic love affair" (Pintilie 2015:130). If she has Louis to herself, Claudia believes he is content with her, never fearing that she will lose him. However, after he meets with a community of vampires in Paris, she realizes that she does not belong in this select world, meaning her hold on to Louis is tenuous, at best. As a vampire, she still needs Louis's protection from the Paris vampires, who see her as a threat. Because he senses Claudia is in danger, Louis goes to see Armand, the leader of the vampires in Paris, the man who wants to be Louis's lover. Substantiating Louis' fears, Armand states, "I will give you reasons, her silence, her youth. It is forbidden to make one so young, so helpless that it cannot survive on its own". (*Interview with the* Vampire) With the mind and heart of a woman in love, Claudia knows that her time with Louis is now over. Simultaneously, Claudia realizes the finality of her relationship with Louis, accepting that she cannot exist without him. It is more than a matter of the heart; it is also practicality. She needs Louis to survive physically. This is the tragedy of Claudia; her body is her prison, which is why she cannot live. Claudia's tragic death at the hands of the Paris vampires is heartbreakingly horrific yet, most of all, unfortunately inevitable.

Interview with the Vampire (2023) AMC Networks

The most current iteration of Rice's work is the new *Interview with the Vampire* series on AMC Networks. Although this version of Rice's work has been controversial, it is not about casting but instead about deviations from the novel. The series is set in New Orleans, but the time period has been moved up to the early twentieth century, with Louis as a black brothel owner. Additionally, the series does not just make one bold move but two by turning Claudia into a biracial character. Again, this changes the whole image of Claudia, giving her another dimension.

In the series, Louis finds Claudia in a burning building after a race riot. She is 14, portrayed by 19-year-old Bailey Bass. Again, the difficulty of filming this story lies within the apparent contradictions in depicting a mentally maturing Claudia evolving over the years as an adult while dealing with her never-changing adolescent appearance. Acknowledging that Claudia is a teenager who will never physically evolve into an adult woman, this series aims to illustrate her as the "average teenager" who happens to be a vampire. She has a diary, a first love, and goes on a sojourn to college, but everything is complicated by being a vampire. Yet, this version of Claudia is unlike the others because she is "turned" at 14 and thinks about her identity from the perspective of who she was and what she has become. However, similar to the other versions of Claudia, her acquiescence of her vampire nature isimmediate. So much so that Louis and Lestat must teach her that she cannot pursue her every whim. Emphatically, Lestat instructs her on the art of killing.

Claudia's realization of her stunted growth comes to fruition when Lestat takes her to lovers' lane, his favorite hunting ground. Lestat urges her to go in for the kill as they watch the kids making out. Reminiscent of Claudia's recognition scene with the Creole woman in the film, in the series, before Claudia jumps on the couple, she is somewhat hypnotized by the view of the naked girl. She is mesmerized by the girl as she sees what she is not. Even though Claudia is now 18, she is fully aware of the striking difference between the girl's look and her appearance. She does not ask questions but pounces on the girl with the ardency of a killer, probably because she wants to destroy what she cannot be. Claudia can never be what she was (human) because, as scholar Winnbust points out, "the vampire pollutes all systems of kinship, pollutes all systems of blood, pollutes all systems of race and sex and desire that must be straight. He infects the body and thereby *alters the spirit*--nobody can transcend the metamorphoses of his bite..." (Winnubst 2003:8). Lestat's bite has changed forever the world Claudia previously knew because now she has been transformed into the killer. Regardless, Claudia cannot hold onto her old life. She cannot transcend the change; she must submit.

The television series made another significant change to Claudia's character, and that was to tone down the sexuality issue. They aged her to 14, but at least during the first season, they make it clear that her relationship with Louis is one of father/daughter. To a significant degree, that deviation halts some of the issues that have plagued her character since its creation. Specifically, Claudia's sexuality is limited to outside her created vampire family. The new iteration of Claudia has neutered one of the most controversial aspects of her character. Of course, the show did this because it must continue on a series renewal basis so the character cannot crash and burn.

In conclusion, from the beginning of her literary debut in *Interview with the Vampire*, Claudia presented a duality that transcended while transforming the mythical/legendary world of horror inhabited by vampires. Caught between the raging conflicts of existing as a child vampire, physical immutability versus psychological growth, Claudia becomes the object of a latent ambiguous depiction of sexuality in a child. Whether Claudia is five, ten, or fourteen, she is constrained by having to live eternally in a childhood/teenage space. Anne Rice created a character who shifts boundaries of age, mental maturity, and agency. When discussing vampires and aging, one must deal with the fact that many people would love immortality because it would mean they would never have to grow old. The construct of immortality must include youth, or it is not wanted. Most people would not want immortality if they had to deal with being an elderly person for eternity. But the reverse is true for Claudia. For Claudia, youth and immortality are her problems. Imprisoned by her eternal youth, her endowment of immortality lacks agency or empowerment. Her tragedy is not just that she will never grow up but that she first had her mortal life taken without her consent. Secondly, she cannot exist without other vampires – dependent forever on them for survival. Additionally, in her visual depictions, dealing with her sexuality is still very controversial because of her childlike image. Claudia can never be fully a woman because vampires and human society will always see her as a child. She was not meant to stay in the vampire world, especially Rice's; it is a challenge for a woman to survive in Anne Rice's masculine universe. Under the spell of Rice's masterful literary skills, the reader travels along obligingly in the path of Claudia's fierce determination to overcome the obstacles of her stunted physicality and her lack of the defining element: the vampire's ability to defy death.

Author Bio

I am Dr. Kimberly Smith, Assistant Professor of English at Elizabeth City State University. I received my BA from Georgia State University, MA from Rutgers University, and Doctorate from SUNY at Stony Brook. My dissertation is entitled *Gothic Elements and Racial Stereotypes in the Construction of the Passing Character*. My areas of research and study are American Literature, Gothicism, and Popular Culture, with an emphasis on television. I am in the process of writing a book on the representation of single women on television which is in the revision stage. I also have an essay entitled. "The World War II Christmas: Gender and Class *Christmas in Connecticut* (1945) and *It Happened on 5th Avenue* (1947) in the forthcoming anthology entitled *Under the Mistletoe: Essays on Holiday Romance in Popular Culture.*

Works Cited

Fenn, Violet (2021): A History of the Vampire in Popular Culture: Love at First Bite, Philadelphia: Pen and Sword History.
Haynes, Todd (2023): May December. Netflix
Horner, Avril and Zlosnik, Sue (2016): "No Country for Old Women: Gender, Age and the Gothic." In: Avril Horner Sue Zlosnik (eds), Women and The Gothic an Edinburgh Companion, Edinburgh: Edinburgh University Press, pgs. 185–196.
Jordan, Neil (2000): Interview with the Vampire. Warner Brothers.
Jordan, Neil (1997): Commentary. Interview with the Vampire, Warner Brothers.
Jowett, L. (2002): "Mute and Beautiful: The Representation of the Female in Anne Rice's Interview with the Vampire." In: Femspec 3/1, 59.
Le Fanu, Joseph Sheridan (2023): Carmilla, Garret McCarty.
Madalina-Pintilie, Iulia (2015) "Gender Conventions: Homosexual Eroticism and Family Liaisons in Anne Rice and Neil Jordan's Interview with the Vampire." Journal of Romanian Studies 7, 642–652.
McDevitt, Kelly (July 2020) "Childhood Sexuality as Posthuman Subjectivity in Octavia E. Butler's Fledgling." Science Fiction Studies, 46/2, 219–240.
Shakespeare William "Hamlet" In Martin Puchner and Suzanne Akbari and Wiebke Denecke and Barbara Fuchs and Caroline Levine and Pericles Lewis and Emily Wilson (eds), The Norton Anthology of World Literature: Shorter Fourth Edition Volume 1, New York: W.W. Norton, pp. 1708–1809.
Ramsland, Katherine (2010): Prism of the Night: A Biography of Anne Rice, New York: Random House.
Reep, Diana C. and J Ceccio, Joseph F. Ceccio and Francis, William A (1996) "Anne Rice's Interview with the Vampire: Novel versus Film" In Gary Happenstand and Ray B. Browne(eds), The Gothic World of

Anne Rice, Bowling Green, Oh: Bowling State Green Popular Press, 123–148.

Rice, Anne (1997) Interview with the Vampire, New York: Ballantine.

Waxman, Barbara Fray "Post existentialism in the Neo-Gothic Mode: Anne Rice's Interview with The Vampire." (Summer 1992) Mosaic: An Interdisciplinary Critical Journal, 25/3, pp. 70–97.

Winnubst, Shannon. (Fall 2003) "Vampires, Anxieties, and Dreams: Race and Sex in the Contemporary United States." Hypatia, 18/3, pp. 1–20.

Childhood at the Center
The Horror of Miles and Flora in Henry James's
The Turn of the Screw (1898) and Jack Clayton's
Film Adaptation *The Innocents* (1961)

Vitor Alves Silva[1]

> "*Schizoid* behavior is a pretty common thing in children. It's accepted, because all [...] adults have this unspoken agreement that children are lunatics."
> (King 1977: 114)

Children as Children

Although for any contemporary academic working with James's *oeuvre*, it'd be hard to completely dismiss the role childhood and, more specifically, the characters of Miles and Flora, play in *The Turn of the Screw*, it's evident that their utilization as mere stepping stones in the service of grander hermeneutical pursuits is far from a rare occurrence. The primary efforts of scholars of the novella tend to shift between the psychosexual Freudian reading anchored in the psychological state of the adult characters, particularly the governess, and the metaphysical aspect associated with the reality of the occurring supernatural events. Though

---

1 University of Porto.

childhood is often at play in both of these approaches, the aforementioned characters tend towards utilization as complements more than as the narrative axioms they can be considered, if one but acknowledges how transversally present they've been in the original work and subsequent adaptations.

The tendency of academic literature to read Miles and Flora as elements of supplementation instead of causation has led me to believe that even though research around *The Turn of the Screw* has recognized the importance of the narrative interplays the characters offer, it has been rather insufficient in properly articulating the paramount role they have in dictating and influencing other characters' actions and motivations. This realization is the root for the titular article, which aims to dialogue with other texts in the now-expanding conversation about the centrality of childhood in the narrative, via the proposal of a mode of reading that classifies Miles and Flora as the hermeneutical centers, therefore challenging the prevailing viewpoints that relegate them to peripheral analytical roles in this context. I aim to illustrate that they can constitute the interpretative focus independently of the interpretative approach one adheres to, by shedding light on the key mechanisms through which they (and childhood *stricto sensu*) are present and reverberate on other textual narrative elements.

Believing *The Innocents*, directed by Jack Clayton, to be the adaptation which best illustrates this connection to childhood, by virtue, for example, of its title (which denotes its focus on childish innocence), I aim also to cross-read it with James's novella, and offer a comprehensive contextualization of some of the themes introduced by the presence of Miles and Flora in both works. I wish to treat the child characters as children and, ultimately, I aim to prove that they allow for the existence of narrative dichotomies of innocence/sexuality and child/adult power dynamics, effectively surging on the narrative its most important elements of uneasiness, ambiguity, horror, moral panic and perversion.

To many readers, the most important aspect of the original novella, which also evidently translates into the titular adaptation, is its deliberate ambiguity. Douglas and the governess are seen as its major contributors because they infuse the narrative with their subjective perspectives and biases. Douglas, as the primary narrator, serves as the intermediary between the reader and the written account of the governess. While he presents himself as an authoritative figure, possessing the manuscript that serves as textual basis and recounting the story to his attentive audience, his own motivations and biases come into question; his interpretation and retelling of the events inevitably shape the reader's understanding, introducing an element of uncertainty and subjectivity. Douglas's role as a storyteller and his privileged position means the governess's account is *washed through* his thoughts and words. The readers are left to question his reliability, wondering whether he may be embellishing or interpreting the account, and what implications this may have for the overall reception of textual information. This choice of structure allows for a layered storytelling approach, but also perceivably distances the reader from direct engagement with the children.

Similarly, the governess herself emerges as an unreliable narrator, due to her increasingly obsessive behavior towards the perceived malevolent influence of the ghosts, blurring the boundaries between reality and imagination. As a central figure in the story, she serves as the primary conduit through which the events unfold, creating what appears to be an even deeper disconnection to what this paper proposes. It is through this deliberate ambiguity that Henry James masterfully crafts a narrative that transcends a straightforward ghost story; both Douglas's and the governess's untrustworthiness act as endlessly fascinating invitations to debate, allowing the novella to still constitute itself as a fertile ground for different academic pursuits. Even if the acknowledgement of Miles and Flora's narrative importance isn't necessarily incompatible with the importance of both of these characters (I'm not adopting an essentialist stance on interpretation), can their hermeneutic centrality be defended?

However totalizing and satisfactory these observations seem to be in accounting for the element of ambiguity, one must consider that the governess only comes to constitute herself as unreliable due to her intense focus on the children and their protection. Her supernatural conundrum stems from the necessity to shield the pure innocence of Miles and Flora from the hints of sexuality, corruption or possession associated with the spirits. Their actions and interactions with the governess become pivotal moments that shape her psychological journey – and therefore, any assumption of the governess as the central hermeneutic element realistically underlies the assumption of Miles and Flora's evident narrative reverberations. Her self-imposed duty is not only central to her character's existence; it is the baseline, relentless and most stable building block when considering her presentation, actions and thoughts. Her fixation permeates every aspect of her existence, as she admits to "overscoring their full hours" (James 2008: 43). Literary critic Shoshanna Felman (qtd. in Hanson 2021: 249), highlights the way *The Turn of the Screw* turns readers, especially those with a psychoanalytic perspective, into governesses who become suspicious of the sexual secrets of the children themselves; effectively arguing for the children's centrality to the reader experience. Douglas, in turn, recognizes the children's central importance in the story immediately in the prologue, when mentioning the metaphorical connection between the act of "turning the screw" and the vanguardist insertion of childhood characters in a report about spiritism filled to the brim with sexual undertones. Describing this section of the original novella, English literature expert Tydal writes:

> After one particularly spine-tingling tale, involving a young boy awakened by an apparition, the friends agree that ghost stories where children play a prominent part are the most chilling; the presence of little ones in the face of the spectral, as it is put, provides 'another turn of the screw.' Much to the delight of everyone present, one of the men in the party announces that he also knows a story falling under this category. What is more, not only is the story allegedly true, but it also has the added attraction of involving two children – giving 'two turns' to that same screw. The story the man proceeds to tell then becomes the story we are reading, as the governess proceeds to take up her position at Bly House. While the prologue does not necessarily attribute monstrous agency to the children, it does suggest that their role in the story is central to the reader's experience of horror. (Tydal 2015: 192)

Miles and Flora can easily be considered the root cause of ambiguity in the novel through association with other thematic dichotomies, mainly class transgression and sexually improper behavior. Mrs. Grose's revelation of a hinted sexual connection between the valet Quint and Miles hints at not only a class conflict but one of (homo)sexuality and depravedness. It seems that they are, indeed, inescapable, and in Clayton's *The Innocents*, this argument is even more sustainable, as the paranormal elements are introduced before the idea of the governess's unreliability. Shortly after her arrival at Bly, the governess witnesses Flora "humming the vaguely eerie song 'O Willow Waley', as if a mystical summons" (ibid: 194) and, "at this point in the film, the viewer has little reason to believe that anything is afoul at Bly, since no ghosts have yet appeared. [...] In other words, we are introduced to the idea of the potentially monstrous children before the idea of the potentially insane governess" (ibid). Considering this very promising landscape, the centrality of childhood in the novella seems like a delicious proposition.

Transgressive Fantasies: Childhood, Innocence and Sexuality

It'd be impossible to refer to the story's themes without referring, primarily, its emphasis on innocence. Though not a lot has been written about the novella in a perspective that privileges its child characters, most of the scholarly contributions in this regard tend to lean heavily on the concept. Literary scholar James Kincaid, with his work *Erotic Innocence* (1998) is one of the biggest contributors to this conversation, bridging the themes that give this chapter its title.

In his work, Kincaid, referring to the original novella, emphasizes three crucial aspects of its innocent child characters. Firstly, he argues that Miles and Flora's innocence is not something inherent or discovered but rather shaped by norms and expectations; a "concocted" process (2021: 156). This type of process, he defends, is characteristically unnatural in the sense that it's not necessarily biologically dictated, constituting itself primarily as a social advent as opposed to an intrinsic property of the children. Secondly, he notes said innocence is allowed to thrive due to not only being "protected but actively inculcated" (ibid), calling attention to the necessity of enforcement in order to achieve its implementation[2]. Lastly, Kincaid critiques the exaggerated prominence of the concept of innocence during the Victorian era, suggesting that it reveals our own contemporary needs of projecting pureness and injecting it into the figure of the child which is, by itself, a far more complex and often discomforting category (ibid).

What I'd like to argue for, through Kincaid's matrix, is that any attempts to, as he writes, maintain this innocence by enforcing it on behalf of the governess, who conceives it as intrinsic to the children, feeds into a misguided paradox, and end up generating the opposite effect of further corrupting them. I would also like to argue that innocence, as it is portrayed in the novella and the film, is fundamentally paradoxical, as it is by necessity built against and upon its contrary: sexual impulses, sexuality and sexual depravity. Above all, though, I will attempt to defend, mainly referring to Kincaid's arguments about infant sexualization in mainstream media, that Miles and Flora's significance as conductors of James's and Clayton's narratives heavily relies on relations established between childhood, innocence and sexuality as concepts associated to them via the novella's implied Victorian frame of reference.

Firstly, it's easy to notice that both Miles and Flora are weak and fragilized in terms of their susceptibility to external influences: the estate of Bly is rather isolated, and with the death of their parents, any peripheral social interaction apart from the one established with the housemaid Mrs. Grose is sure to be paramount in their upbringing. The two main ideas present in this characterization – a child's influenceability and the lack of a parental figure – are deeply connected to

---

2   In the case of Miles and Flora, this can be best exemplified by the governess's hesitation in acknowledging Miles' wrongdoings as it pertains to his academic expulsion, for example – going so far as to equate him to a divine figure. Schober's analysis very eloquently shows how her perception of the children as unmistakably innocent happens not through cause and effect, but by definition; she sees them as the embodiment of goodness, as "even when [they are] bad, they are good" (Schober 2004: 57).

Victorian literary tropes that permeate James's transitional fin-de-siècle background. Scholar Ben Moore writes that one of the most prominent ways of representing children in Victorian literature deals with "the idealized Romantic child, typically conceived as naturally innocent and close to God" (2017: 1). In her book *The Gothic Child* (2013), child literature researcher Margarita Georgieva also mentions the prominence of orphanhood, claiming that these tropes reflect the anxieties and societal concerns of the time, regarding the breakdown of the traditional family structure in the periods pre-dating the first world war.

As English literature historian Scofield denotes, Miles and Flora's characterization stands in concordance with the ideals of "female purity" and the "unspeakableness of sexuality" (2003: 4). It is the absence of parental figures mentioned by Georgieva which accentuates the children's susceptibility to external forces, and allows for the computing of the supernatural entities in the titular works as perilous and potentially dangerous. At the same time, it's the fear for erosion of traditional family values that calls forth the sexual innuendo associated to the characters of Quint and Miss Jessel – the spectral deviants that would lead them astray from innocence (with innocence and family being directly correlated to religious values of Christian familyhood, moral purity and sexual celibacy). Any act of sexual engagement, even if part of regular development, is posited as outside of the domain of the Christian and Victorian child by default, and therefore considered as corruptive of the child character's innocence.

Whether it's Quint being *too free* or strategic nods to class conflation as a consequence of his and Miss Jessel's relationship, sex is at the basis of the element of corruption associated with the spectral figures. According to child literature researcher Lucija Stambolija, "words that James uses repeatedly throughout the novella [...] are highly allusive of sex: erect (three times), intercourse (five times), perverse, intimately (three times), etc." (2020: 12). It seems, then, that the question of sexuality is unavoidable, even if we don't adhere to the idea that the ghosts are a symbol for the governess's repression of it. As Victorian literature scholar Ellis Hanson denotes, sexuality is also a rather primary element in accounting for reader discomfort and for one's engagement with the narrative. It's an element of connection between our discomfort and the governess's report:

> By proposing that Quint was too free not only with the boy but with 'every one', Mrs. Grose would seem to include not only herself and the governess but also the reader in a pedophilic seduction that knows no limits, as if to seduce a child were to court the essence of seduction itself and implicate even the most casual bystander. There are no innocent readers of this text, it has often been pointed out, but we are infantilized by our very belief in innocence. We feel that our childlike innocent has been imposed on and corrupted by Quint, that we have been made to contemplate matters, specifically sexual matters, that ought to remain safely outside of our ken. (Hanson 2021: 246)

By trying to deliberately shield the children from sexuality (the ghosts – either symbols of child sexualization or echoes of anti-Christian conduct), the governess inevitably draws attention to it as a constitutive axiomatic opposite at every turn, creating what is essentially a paradox of protection that actively undermines its pretenses. If one considers the very concept of childish innocence in the texts, which the governess tries to preserve, as constituted by elements that can only exist when built upon the opposite force of sexuality, it becomes easy to notice that every attempt at preserving innocence is by default counterproductive – it leads Miles and Flora away from Christian, pure values of family and sexual inexistence. Since one could go so far as to say that a lack of sexual engagement/development is a necessary stepping stone in this acceptation of innocence, it becomes possible to argue, even, that the concept of innocence itself, as portrayed in the novella and the film, works as a sort of vacuum, a state of *not-knowing*. It's built by opposition to the expectation of sexual deviancy.

Barnsley, childhood and post-colonial literature expert, demonstrated this effect quite well, by denoting, for example, how the effect of visual representation of child nudity as innocent tends to "have the effect of sexualizing the child through the look" (2010: 328). Though not referring to the titular novella and adaptation, this insight can realistically be called forth in an analysis of either, as the need to enforce innocence inevitably engages and draws attention to its opposite. The forceful framing of children as inherently non-sexual (innocent) in the novella and film implies the existence of a possibly corrupting force – or, in other words, the governess's overprotective tendencies end up calling attention to and conjuring ghosts of sexuality which are consciously repressed.

The argument for the implications traditional Christian values could have in the sexual repression of children as they traverse puberty is appealing in the sense that it's easy. However, I'd instead like to explore the concept of agency, more specifically the governess's agency, in accounting for the corruption of the children. Though the ghosts of Quint and Jessel are perceived as opportunistic in the sense that they'd take advantage of the parentless and influenceable children, how wrong would one be to suggest a similar process is at play with the governess? Not only does she have a significant hold over the children which allows her to assert her more comparatively powerful status (she assumes the role of a parental figure as the children's uncle allows her for full educative freedom), she's also the only real contact with the outside world Miles and Flora enjoy during the duration of the narrative[3]. Keeping in mind that the governess, when compared to the spectral presences of Quint and Jessel, has the same tools for corruption at her disposal, and is attempting to forcefully instate a very specific mode of existence upon the children (Christian values, family, celibacy, asexuality), is a necessity.

In order to talk about the governess's influence on the children, it's important to mobilize once again Barnsley's seminal paper "The Child/ The Future", where the author writes that "the figure of the child often indicates spontaneity, innocence and originality as well as pure simplicity and imitation" (ibid: 323). I particularly wish to focus on the word "imitation" and its employment here. The idea that children learn through imitation is not new. According to Aristotle, as far back as the 5th century BC, human beings have an innate tendency towards imitation, which plays

---

3   There is, eventually, a reference to the nearest village which contains a church. By itself, however, it is insufficient in disproving the point.

a significant role in the formation of their character and understanding of the world (Poética, 1448b5). In the context of innocence, mimesis suggests that children, in their naivety and lack of worldly experience, imitate and reflect the behavior and ideals of those around them. Meltzoff and Moore's imitation study (1977), is a rather elucidating inquiry that points to newborn infants' ability to imitate facial expressions, for example, effectively proving this process of imitation as learning to be, at least to some extent, true. The researchers found that infants as young as 12 to 21 days old could mimic specific facial gestures made by an adult model, which allows for the framing of imitation as a fundamental mechanism for learning during childhood. Equally, Albert Bandura's Bobo Doll experiment (1961) shows how imitative processes can work inversely, allowing for the undertaking of more questionable learnings. In the experiment, children observed an adult model engaging in aggressive behavior towards a doll, and it was found that children who witnessed the aggressive behavior were more likely to imitate it compared to those who did not.

The implication of imitation as an apparatus for learning is clearly something the governess recognizes, as when thinking about the children's previous misbehaviors, alluded to by Mrs. Grose in Chapter IX, she tends to associate them to the ghosts of Quint and Jessel. In framing the ghosts as a malevolent entity that aims to contaminate and pervert the children, the governess seems to posit herself as a worthy alternative for imitation. Flora and Miles are under the spell and she is the one to break it. She regards herself as a pure soul from which to model the children after. At the very least, one can claim she does not believe or is in any way conscious of any elements that would disrupt this perception. Oddly, however, the children never seem to passively absorb her teachings; she has to constantly and forcefully (even violently) compete with the supposed spectral influence through enforced behavior. As critic and essayist Richard Locke puts it, she's constantly "imposing such violent absolutes on [the] children in ways that empower [herself] and destroy children." (2011: 88). Stambolija even goes as far as to note that "while it is rather clear that the governess's idea of the greatest danger to one's innocence is directly related to sexuality, it is not the ghosts who create the gloomy atmosphere that the governess so fears. [...] It is, in fact, the governess 'who instinctively identifies sex with the powers of darkness and evil'. [...] The ghosts themselves remain, as it were, asexual.'" (2010: 14).

How should we go about accounting for this purposeful projection of a sexual nature onto the spectral figures when they do not manifest in any sexual way to the governess? The only possible solution is to consider her morally degraded. Should we adhere to the psychoanalytic reading and identify the ghosts as a manifestation of sexual repression, this position becomes even easier to defend. If the ghosts are, then, a symbol of the consequences of her sexual fantasy with Miles's uncle, which is often hinted at in the novel, then the evident conclusion is that she is neither uncorrupted nor pure – she becomes a wicked model for imitation. Al-Qurani, assistant professor of literature at King Khalid University, writes:

> Miss Jessel, in a psychoanalytic reading of the text, may then exist as a symbolic representation of the desires the governess cannot admit or express. This hallucination has been borne of the governess's dangerous indulgence in sexual fantasies about her employer. Miss Jessel must therefore be detested as evil by a governess seeking to repress her own similar sexual urges. (Al-Qurani 2013: 84)

The idea that she can, as a character, mirror the same amount of impurity and corruption as those she comes to associate with Quint and Miss Jessel is very telling.

It might also be possible to identify, on her part, a sense of erotic fascination towards the children and, in particular, towards Miles, which constitutes an even more evident transgression to his innocence, and an even more immediate parallel with some interpretative approaches to the presence of the ghosts in the narratives. As Schober, expert on childhood in cinema, writes, to the governess, "Miles appears at once innocent and childlike and experienced and adult, which both excites and disturbs her" (2004: 62) – emphasis on "excites". Similarly, as pointed out by Locke, "she is attracted to Miles because he has something divine [...]

as if he had never for a second suffered" and, in the perceived necessity to shelter that holiness, she actively chooses to neglect his tragic reality; "his family history of death and neglect – the deaths of his parents and grandparents and of Jessel and Quint; the many separations and displacements." (2011: 91). The Christian notion of the sanctity of the body, especially the child's body, which is definitely present in the text, while not explicitly erotic, can be seen as inherently charged with sexual undertones, as it focuses attention on the body itself. Similarly, the religious *ethos* of self-sacrifice is evidently twisted in the governess's character, through a process of *quasi-fetishization* of her acts of service in the domains of their education, upbringing and sociality.

A very significant difference between the original novella and Clayton's film are the two kisses the governess exchanges with Miles – both very erotic and on the lips. Though erotic tension in the novella is often present, such as in most of the scenes where Miles refers to the governess as "my dear", it is never as direct as what is shown to us by Clayton. As Stambolija notes, Clayton may simply be pointing towards the fact that "she is in love with Miles's uncle, and that perhaps this infatuation influences her feelings towards the child." (2020: 22). However, in both scenes, it's she who initiates the kissing action, with Miles being but a passive receiver and appearing shocked – be it because of the pervasive sexual intrusion of the situation, or because he is really possessed by the ghost of Peter Quint. Either way, making a case for why her attempts at reinforcing the children's innocence are counterproductive in this interpretative optic becomes rather easy. Similarly, the idea that Miles's and Flora's susceptibility to their environment might be central in the novella becomes ever more appealing. In her 2016 book, *Evil Children in the Popular Imagination*, horror film scholar Karen Renner writes:

> Possession narratives act as cautionary tales that warn viewer, in symbolic terms, that children are vulnerable to dangerous influences when traditional family structures are damaged and parents are negligent in their duties. These texts imply that 'exorcism' requires not merely a formal religious ritual but an entire reconfiguration of the family unit. (Renner 2016: 123)

Equating the governess in the way I have thus far advocated for would imply seeing her as a poor substitute parental figure. Miles and Flora are always central to James's and Clayton's irony: we are introduced to the theme of family value preservation by association with Quint and Jessel, and then he inverts them as it pertains to how he characterizes the governess. The "exorcism" (the expulsion of the entities that hold such a corruptive power of the children) that Renner mentions might find a worthier adversary in the governess than the spectral appearances, especially considering we cannot say for sure whether they are or aren't framed as actually real.

The ultimate argument that can be conjured to support the idea that innocence is indeed constituted practically in relation to sexuality and sexual expression, however, is the one related to Miles's confession. In the novella and film's climax, the governess demands that Miles confesses to having seen Peter Quint, therefore implying the specter to have had some sort of corruptive influence upon him. Whether you adopt the psychosexual interpretation (and therefore assume this confession to mean the corruption of the child through sexual depravity) or the metaphysical one (and therefore assume the sexual innuendo to be directly interlaced with sexual development and maturation), if Miles confessed, he would be breaking his *façade* of innocence regardless. Though she asks him to confess in an ultimate grand act – a big final attempt at the preservation of his innocence, a saving of the soul – if he obeys, he is doomed never to go back to untarnished innocence. By staying silent, he passively engages in the governess's fantasy of ghostly influence, which will cause her to classify him as being over the point of salvation, considering how convinced of the reality of possession she seems by the end of the novella. By speaking, he confesses to having been influenced, and *knowing* (both literally and figuratively, or even in a biblical sense) sexual deviancy. Miles cannot go back to being innocent because wanting to do so implies knowing what is and isn't innocent; and to distinguish between the two makes for the impossibility of forgetting said distinction. To know what innocence isn't is to automatically stop being innocent, and not being able to return. As Hanson writes, "Such innocence always bears in its logic of purity the fantasy of its own violation, the fantasy that sustains it and shatters it at the same time. It must perform itself without knowing itself, since, for a child, to understand the meaning of innocence is to already have lost it." (2021: 252).

Monster Children: Childhood, Normativity and the Uncanny

> 'Master Miles is a good boy,' Mrs. Grose almost pleads with her, 'there's nothing wicked in him.' To this, the governess retorts: 'Unless he's deceiving us; unless they're both deceiving us', after which she stops for a second, to then carefully articulate: 'The innocents ...' The delivery of the line is striking: it is as if the governess realizes the irony of what she is saying at the moment she speaks it. Standing out due to its invocation of the film's title, the comment goes to the very heart of the difference between the novella and Clayton's adaptation, namely how it shifts the weight of titillating ambiguity from the insanity of the governess to the monstrosity of the children. In doing so, *The Innocents* also opens up a site of potential horror that was indeed present in the original tale, but which had been obscured by the polarization of the critical debate: the secret world of childhood. (Tydal 2015: 196–197)

In both the film and the novella, the idea of a *secret world of childhood* plays a significant role in evoking discomfort and fear for both the governess and the readers. The idea of a *secret world* as it pertains to childhood denotes an inherent incomprehension of what said world entails, and not understanding the children is inevitably a source of discomfort for the governess, as it furthers her possible paranoia with regard to the spectral influence the ghosts hold over them. It becomes important, then, to explore the elusiveness of Miles and Flora's actions, situating them in said *unknown world*, arguing for it as a point of liberation, autonomy and escapism which stands opposed to the governess's tyrannical impositions. I will try to show how prevalent the ideas of occultation and absence are in the construction of several narrative devices, and how they're usually products of Miles and Flora's central hermeneutical presence, essentially contributing to the most notable axiom of James's original novella: its interpretative ambiguity. Lastly, I will also try to explain why this occultation and absence are elements that classify the children as monsters, and how exactly they come to signify as such.

One pivotal moment highlighting the theme of childhood secrets occurs during a conversation between the governess and the children. When the governess comments on the size of the house, Miles responds by inquiring about her own family home, asking if it was too small for her to have secrets. Unbeknownst to the governess, the children exchange a knowing look. While she fails to grasp the subtext, the implication is clear: the expansive estate of Bly allows the children to maintain their private world, hidden from the prying eyes of adults (ibid: 197). The grand and mysterious estate serves as an ideal setting for the children's privacy; its sheer size and sprawling nature create a physical space that fosters seclusion and hidden corners, shielding them from external intrusions. The vastness of the manor allows for secret spaces and areas they can retreat to and utilize to cultivate their own realm of mystery and intrigue while remaining absent from the governess's general influence. Miles's defiant act of sneaking out during the night, which can be seen as his frustrated attempt at asserting independence and dissociating from the governess's authority, illustrates the umbilical relationship between privacy, misdirection and the sheer size of the estate of Bly. He manages to keep his true intentions hidden because the space physically allows him to do so, which wouldn't have necessarily been possible was he sleeping in the same room as the governess, like Flora. Bly, one could say, by its existence alone, seems to act as a rather central, almost character-like bit of the narrative, as the governess herself remarks on its magnitude, highlighting its capacity to hold numerous hidden secrets within its walls: "Was there a 'secret' at Bly- a mystery of Udolpho or an insane, an unmentionable relative kept in unsuspected confinement?" (James 2008: 21). By giving the children a space where their intentions and motives remain shrouded in mystery, the estate not only amplifies the governess's uncertainty about the children's innocence, it also impedes the reader of fully deciphering their true nature, which both intrigues and horrifies her. It manages to keep absent what would otherwise be present. Clayton's film, by deliberately dipping substantial parts of the house in darkness, as if hiding from possible spectators that which is also outside of the governess's sway, can spawn even more examples.

Secrets and occultation of information often end up acting as twisted confirmation. Faced with this absence, the governess's reaction becomes exacerbated to the point of no return. As Schober mentions, "the apparitions themselves function as blank pages upon which meaning is inscribed" (2004: 60). Similarly, the process through which information is hidden as it pertains to Miles and Flora's doing allows the governess a platform for projection of her wants and needs. She interprets the possible spectral presences as a confirmation of evil. Likewise, the possessed children's unnatural goodness is defined through the absence of sexual deviancy, which suggests the potential for evil to occupy them – once she loses confidence in Flora's innocence, interpreting her silence as a sign that she is under the influence of the malevolent Miss Jessel, the emptiness of the child is filled with the knowledge of impurity. The limited insight into the children's private world parallels her tendency to want to be integrally aware of the children's every dimension and, at the same time, her sheer inability to perceive childhood as anything more than mere inherent innocence.

Absence of innocence is also communicated through the vessel of Bly and through the idea of occultation and secrecy. One of the unsettling aspects of the novella, for example, is the children's ability to speak in a manner that surpasses their expected age and experience. Miles's use of the term "my dear" (found aplenty in chapter XVII) to address the governess is particularly noteworthy, and though it is reverberated in scenes outside of Bly manor, it keeps mostly to one-on-one interactions inside the confines of said space. This endearing way of addressing the other, typically associated with adult discourse, creates a disconcerting effect by blurring the boundaries between childhood innocence and adult familiarity, defying and undermining the traditional power dynamics one would expect between children and adult, and also, clearly challenging the governess's assumed authority by problematizing the reductive categorization of the child as inherently innocent which she tends to enforce. It works on the basis of its assumed instability; Miles utilizes it just enough to arouse suspicion and ambiguity for the reader and the governess, but never fully transgresses into the realm of the unnatural. This blurring of boundaries disrupts our understanding of the children's mental and emotional states, effectively problematizing any monolithic approach to childhood as a category.

The concept of language extends beyond the children's verbal expressions, touching also on the significance of silence in the narrative. Schober, mentions that "one possible sign of Flora's and Miles's corruption is their use of shocking language, the apparent reason for the latter's dismissal from school. (2004: 58). The hinted taboo nature of his possible homosexual proclivity (he only says things to 'Those [he] liked, – James 2008: 90) is underscored by the emphasis on what is left unsaid. The power of silence and absence is once again exemplified by the governess's belief that the children are being controlled by the spirits of Quint and Miss Jessel. She becomes convinced that the only way to save them is to make them confess and utter the names of their tormentors. The act of speaking, of breaking the silence, holds the potential to confront and banish the malevolent forces that possess them. Language, in this context, becomes a tool to combat the unspoken and to restore order – it becomes paramount to the construction of the concepts of confession and control that permeate both the novella and the titular film.

A major tension point of the novella comes from the profound sense of not being able to fully understand the children's mental states. As we delve into the narrative, we often encounter the notion that odd behavior is forgivable in the light of more normalized child behavior. This is significant as it shows that we're used to the trespassing of rational behavior by children, and we've made peace with the idea that the inherent strangeness of children's actions elicits a dual response from adults. When children are perceived as *just being children*, there is a certain allure in observing the inner workings of their minds. It's as if they inhabit a realm that transcends conventional understanding. However, this fascination is equally tempered by the disconcerting notion of *not-knowing*, of never being able to fully grasp the depths of their thoughts and motivations. This tension – a mixture of fascination and horror – is explored repeatedly in the novella and is what transmutes the children from tangible, innocent beings into something more sinister and mysterious, even demonic:

> He [Miles] sat down at the old piano and played as he had never played; and if there are those who think he had better have been kicking a football I can only say that I wholly agree with them. For at the end of a time that under his influence I had quite ceased to measure, I started up with a strange sense of having literally slept at my post. (James 2008: 111)

The truly terrifying aspect of this scenario is that Miles's capacity for destruction is limited only by his inherent helplessness. The children's actions are curtailed by the natural constraints of childhood, where they rely on adults for supervision, guidance, and protection. Their lack of physical strength or independence is what often keeps their potentially harmful desires in check. However, the heart of the horror lies in the idea of removing this helplessness. If you take away the restraints that naturally limit the actions of children, you unleash the potential of an unmeasurable power. As such, the idea of the children being endowed with an extremely high level of communication, connivance, verbosity or even musical proficiency makes it so we can no longer set rational boundaries, which turns Miles and Flora into a very powerful source of fear and discomfort.

The concept of the *uncanny valley*, albeit originated in the field of robotics, offers an interesting matrix in this context. It was usually utilized to refer to the discomfort or eeriness that people often experienced when they encountered a humanoid robot or animated character that closely resembled a human but fell just short of achieving true human-likeness; the idea brought forth by this notion is that as an entity becomes more human-like, our emotional response to it becomes increasingly positive and empathetic. However, there comes a point where the likeness is almost perfect but not quite, and at that juncture, our response turns negative, eliciting a sense of unease, repulsion, or even fear. Miles and Flora, as characters, evoke what could be described as a sense of the uncanny valley – they are human, and yet, their behavior and demeanor deviate ever so slightly from what is expected of children. The novella carefully positions them in this unsettling space, where their actions and speech are just off-kilter enough to create an eerie and disconcerting effect. Arguably, this effect is transversally present across children, turning Miles and Flora into a sort of mirror for the instability of childhood as a category. *The Turn of the Screw* and *The Innocents* both take on the burden of exposing the uncanny nature of childhood by further suggesting that the inherent instability of that category is in itself unsettling; they tease and play with the notion that, due to it lying at the intersection of innocence and the unknown, of what is understood and what remains hidden, childhood is, in and of itself, often scary to adults.

When we consider the entirety of this chapter, it becomes evident how Miles and Flora assume a symbolic significance akin to our cultural imaginaries' monstrous figures, stemming from enduring literary and cinematic creatures that have intrigued and fascinated through similar mechanisms. Just as possessed characters like Regan in William Peter Blatty's *The Exorcist* (1971) are imbued with the horrors of a turbulent coming-of-age, Miles and Flora, too, symbolize a transition of the sort. They share common ground with such archetypal creatures as vampires and werewolves, often depicted as more susceptible to external influences and less adept at navigating complex moral choices, rendering them at the same time vulnerable to and a risk to those around them. Much like the classic Jekyll and Hyde archetype, they even embody the notion that the purity of childhood can swiftly give way to darker impulses and behaviors, underscoring an essentialist view of the dualistic nature of humanity.

In essence, Miles and Flora can indeed be perceived as *the two little monsters*, and Miles's plausible homosexuality further reinforces this claim, as for many individuals within our shared English-language culture, homosexuality was historically regarded as a monstrous condition. "Like an Evil Mr. Hyde, or the Wolfman, a gay [...] self inside you might be striving to get out." (Benshoff 1997: 1). In fact, literature of the Victorian era is rife with examples of monstrous themes that can be examined through a queer lens, from Le Fanu's depiction of the lesbian vampire seductress in *Carmilla* (2005) to the complex secret homosocial relationship in *The Strange Case of Dr. Jekyll and Mr. Hyde* (2003) to Mary Shelley's *Frankenstein* (2003), with its theme's tangents to gender subversions and bodily transformations. Ultimately, Miles and Flora are in concordance with their monster contemporaries in their symbolic status, and remind us that within the supposed innocence of childhood lies a deep well of ambiguity, a space where the line between the familiar and the other blurs.

> It is somewhat analogous to the moment of hesitation that demarcates Todorov's Fantastic, or Freud's theorization of the Uncanny: queerness disrupts narrative equilibrium and sets in motion a questioning of the status quo and, in many cases within fantastic literature, the nature of reality itself." (Benshoff 1997: 5)

Final Remarks

In conclusion, Henry James's *The Turn of the Screw* and its film adaptation, *The Innocents*, directed by Jack Clayton, can be read as primarily an inquiry into the intricate themes of Victorian innocence, sexuality, and the enigmatic nature of childhood existence. Central to both the novella and the film are the roles of Miles and Flora, through which the governess can constitute her narrative significance. The presence of the children as central figures in any interpretation of the narrative highlights their agency and autonomy, urging us to consider their perspectives and motivations, as well as problematizing their power dynamics, their uncanny demeanor and their sophistication in language – all of which resist simple categorization.

By embracing the enigmatic nature of childhood, exploring the repressed themes of sexuality, and placing the central focus on the complex characters of Miles and Flora, the titular objects continue to captivate audiences, provoking thought and inviting us to question our assumptions about how we acknowledge and interact with children. Ultimately, the exploration of the intratextual and intertextual dichotomies of innocence/sexuality and child/adult power dynamics effectively illustrates the significance these characters, as well as the concept of childhood, surge on the narrative and the production of its elements of uneasiness, ambiguity, horror, moral panic and perversion. Both works illuminate the limitations of human understanding of the child, serving as a poignant reminder that the human experience is multifaceted and inherently ambiguous, while defying the status of Miles and Flora as mere *children characters* and instead opting for a more complete characterization which mirrors the inherent monstrosity and uncanny elements transversal to childhood and to its horror media representations.

Author Bio

Vítor Alves Silva is a visual artist, researcher, and curator. His primary research focuses on cinema studies and adaptation processes between literature and cinema, though he often writes on tangent issues pertaining to intermedial studies in general. He maintains a personal interest in side projects encompassing queer and women's themes as well as classical literature.

Works Cited

Al-Qurani, Shonayfa Mohammed (2013):"Hallucinations or Realities: The Ghosts in Henry James's The Turn of the Screw", In: CSCanada Studies in Literature and Language, 6/2, pp. 81–87.
Aristotle (2016): Poética. (E. d. Sousa, Trans.) Lisboa: INCM – Imprensa Nacional Casa da Moeda.

Bandura, Albert/Ross, Dorothea/Ross, Sheila (1961): "Transmission of aggression through imitation of aggressive models", In: Journal of Abnormal and Social Psychology 63, pp. 575–582.
Barnsley, Veronica (2010): "The child/the future", In: Feminist Theory 11/3, pp. 323–330.
Benshoff, Harry (1997): Monsters in the Closet: Homosexuality and the Horror Film. Manchester: Manchester University Press.
Blatty, William Peter (1971): The Exorcist. New York: Harper & Row.
Clayton, Jack (Director), (1961): The Innocents [Motion Picture].
Georgieva, Margarita (2013): The Gothic Child, New York: Palgrave Macmillan.
Hanson, Ellis (2021), "Screwing with Children in Henry James", In: Henry James/Jonathan Warren (Ed.), The Turn of the Screw: Third Norton Critical Edition, New York: Norton & Company, pp. 244–252.
Hitchcock, Alfred (Director), (1954): Rear Window [Motion Picture].
James, Henry (2008): The Turn of the Screw and Other Stories, (Timothy Lustig, Ed.) Oxford: Oxford University Press.
Kincaid, James (1998): Erotic Innocence: The Culture of Child Molesting, Durham: Duke University Press.
Kincaid, James (2021): "Pure and Strangely Erotic: The Victorian Child." In: Henry James/Jonathan Warren (Ed.), The Turn of the Screw: Third Norton Critical Edition, New York: Norton & Company, pp. 153–161.
King, Stephen (1977): The Shining, New York: Doubleday.
Le Fanu, Joseph Sheridan (2005): Carmilla, Maryland: Wildside Press.
Locke, Richard (2011): The Use of Childhood in Ten Great Novels, New York: Columbia University Press.
Maurier, Daphne du (2003): Rebecca, London: Virago.
Meltzoff, Andrew/Moore, Keith (1977): "Imitation of facial and manual gestures by human neonates", In: Science 198, pp. 75–78.
"Childhood in Victorian Literature" by Moore, Ben, May 24, 2017 https://www.oxfordbibliographies.com/display/document/obo-9780199799558/obo-9780199799558-0144.xml
Renner, Karen (2016): Evil Children in the Popular Imagination, New York: Palgrave Macmillan.

Schober, Adrian (2004): Possessed Child Narratives in Literature and Film: Contrary States, New York: Palgrave Macmillan.

Scofield, Martin (2003): "Implied stories: implication, moral panic and the turn of the screw", In: Journal of the Short Story in English 40, pp. 97–107.

Shelley, Mary (2003): Frankenstein. London: Penguin Classics.

Stambolija, Lucija (2020): The Notion of Innocence in Henry James's The Turn of the Screw, Retrieved from Repository of the University of Rijeka, Faculty of Humanities and Social Sciences, September 18, 2020 https://repository.ffri.uniri.hr/islandora/object/ffri:2567

Stevenson, Robert Louis (2003): The Strange Case of Dr. Jekyll and Mr. Hyde and Other Tales of Terror, London: Penguin Classics.

Tydal, Fredrik (2015): "Bringing Out Henry James's Little Monsters: Two Film Approaches to The Turn of the Screw", In: Markus Bohlmann/ Sean Moreland (Eds.), Monstrous Children and Childish Monsters: Essays on Cinema's Holy Terrors, Jefferson: McFarland & Company, Inc., Publishers, pp. 188–209.

Welles, Orson (Director), (1941): Citizen Kane [Motion Picture].

Old Age and Disability as Alterity
Ghosts, (Constructions of) Normalcy and Reliability in *The Others*

Mariana Castelli-Rosa[1]

The Others (2001) is not a typical ghost story: while the film creates the sense of an obvious looming threat, the viewing audience doesn't know the truth about the ghosts during most of the film. This is one of the many deliberate uncertainties of the plot, which lead spectators to make assumptions about which characters represent the otherness referred to by the film's title. By first situating the audience within this uncertainty, the film uses societal expectations and biases to mislead its spectators in their attempts to identify the threat. The main force of the film centers on the servants (two older people and one person with a disability), making them the locus of danger by portraying them as potential threats to the nuclear family because they are old and disabled. The final twists of the film expose this ageist and ablest bias by revealing that all the characters are ghosts, making them all the *real* others of the title, haunting a living family that inhabits the house. All these surprises are possible because of the many uncertainties of the plot play with societal biases, alterity, the abject, and narrative reliability.

In this chapter, I argue that the uncertainties of the plot lead viewers to believe that the threat is located in the older and disabled servants because old age and disability are presented as alterities to the able and young bodies of the members of the Stewart family and because these

---

1   Trent University.

alterities are well-known tropes in the film industry often used to elicit fear in horror films. For this purpose, in addition to studying the portrayals of the three servants and the cultural meanings of old age and disability, I will analyze *The Others* in the context of the genre of horror and ghost stories. I will also touch on narrative (un)reliability and how it increases fear in this film. My objective is to understand how the framing of old age and disability as so-called monstrosities successfully distracts Grace from accessing her memory of what she has done to herself and to her children thus obscuring the real horrors that have happened in her house.

The Others tells the story of Grace Stewart, a woman living in a mansion on the island of Jersey with her two children, Anne and Nicholas. The year is 1945, and she is waiting for her husband to return from the war. As the film begins, three servants arrive. They are: Mrs. Bertha Mills, Mr. Edmund Tuttle and Lydia. Grace believes they are answering an advertisement she had placed in a newspaper after her previous servants suddenly disappeared, but she soon realizes that the letter she wrote to the newspaper looking for help was never sent. Then, strange things start to happen in the house, such as locked doors being unexplainably unlocked and Grace hearing voices in empty rooms. While the servants seem harmless at first and Grace initially welcomes them in the house, as the film progresses, she becomes increasingly suspicious of the three servants and their intentions. As the film is framed to Grace's perspective, viewers are led to likewise doubt the benevolence of the newcomers and believe that they may represent a threat to the family and the house. However, in the midst of this chaos, Anne accuses her mother of being mad and seems to be afraid of her, which hints at the unreliableness of Grace's narrative perspective. Finally, the audience learns that Grace, her children, *and* the servants are all ghosts. These revelations are a shocking reversal for both the family and the film's audience, but the real horror lies in the revelation that Grace was the one who killed her children before killing herself.

Scholar Aviva Briefel considers ghost stories to be a subgenre of horror and places the narrative of *The Others* in the subgenre of "spectral incognizance" (2009: 95), because some of the characters lack knowledge about their status as dead people. Briefel's understanding that ghost stories and horror films have features in common is useful here because the fear and repugnance found in horror films and ghost stories stems from a similar source, that is, the abject. Julia Kristeva classifies the abject as a "threat" (1982: 1), which, in concrete terms, encompasses that which is expelled from the body to protect its boundaries and to, more abstractly, maintain a notion of "identity, system, order" (ibid.: 4). More than something repugnant, the abject disturbs the sense of self exactly because of this ambiguity of its borders in which the self is "in the process of becoming an other" (Kristeva 1982: 3). In other words, the presence of the abject suggests that the body's boundaries are being violated because it is impossible to get rid of its inherent, undesired features.

When it comes to horror films and ghost stories, the abject is linked to the presence of the supernatural because it elicits fear and/or disgust. In *The Others*, particularly, the abject is obvious in the figure of the ghosts that trespass the boundaries of the living and the dead. Moreover, ghosts are "embodied" by dead people and death is the ultimate abject according to Kristeva: "[i]t is death infecting life" (1982: 4). The abjection of ghosts transforms them into an otherness that defies logic (Smajić 2010: 25) and for this reason, creates chaos. In the film, this defiance of logic is obvious in the presence of ghosts, which are not entities most people encounter in their everyday lives. Moreover, the defiance of logic is also apparent in the lack of consistency in the realm of ghosts: Grace has a mirror reflection, but her husband doesn't, for instance. Lastly, the defiance of logic is mirrored in the uncertainties of the plot. Especially of interest here is how the film prompts the audience to resolve all matters of logic by focusing on and magnifying the culturally-sanctioned abjection of bodies of the servants by portraying them as the menace.

The trope of older people as threats is not uncommon. In fact, the use of this trope in cultural productions echoes the belief that the aging of populations is dangerous as seen in the gray tsunami rhetoric and the fear it produces. Similarly, disabled bodies are often used to elicit fear in horror films. These tropes utilize stereotypes that equate old age and disability with a literal embodiment of a deviation from what is considered "normal." These stereotypes are charged with negative connotations in cultural productions, especially in ghost stories and horror films, which appeal to their audience's feelings of fear and disgust. The horror genre's fascination with so-called physical abnormalities, visible to its audiences, emphasizes the human body as a source of fear (Sutton 2017: 73). The so-called abnormality of these bodies is equated with an exposure of undesirable and fear-inducing inner features, an inner evil or menace that would be otherwise hidden from view (Chivers and Markotić 2010: 2; Davis 2016: 9). In *The Others*, disability and old age are framed by the narrative structure of the film to be read as corroboration that the servants are suspicious and threatening. Their dissimilarities to the nuclear family and their abject status as both a part of the household and from outside of the household exacerbate the already present suspicion linked to the servants. This can be seen in the scene where Mrs. Mills tells Anne that "there are going to be big surprises," a line that suggests that the servants have come to the house with an agenda.

Writing about disability and eugenics in the genre of horror, Angela M. Smith states that "the term *monster* deriving from the Latin *monstra*, meaning to show, display or warn, presents aberrant bodies as symbols to be 'read'" (2011: 3). The reading of these bodies-as-symbols doesn't happen in a vacuum. Instead, it is steeped in and mirrors cultural norms, and therefore cultural biases. In the preface of *A Companion to Horror Film*, Harry M. Benshoff explains that "[c]ultural texts such as horror films tell facts about the culture in which they reside: details about gender, about sex, about race and class, about the body, about death, about pain, about being human" (2017: xvi). Cultural symbols and their connotations, positive or negative, already exist within the viewing audience, inscribed by the culture they live in. Viewers bring their expectations about these social signifiers to the films they watch, and likewise, films appeal to the cultural symbols they know the audience brings. As Benshoff explains, the otherness of monsters or of those portrayed as monsters sheds light on what has been deemed undesired in society. Similarly, in *The Horror Film: An Introduction*, Rick Worland explains that the portrayal of monsters or, in this case, ghosts in horror films, gives insight into beliefs in our material world (2007: 13). While horror films may appeal to the metaphysical, they are grounded in our understanding of physical bodies. *The Others* draws parallels between physical bodies that are old or disabled and the monstrous by framing the three servants as scary and/or ill-intentioned. One emblematic scene is when Grace mistrustfully asks Mrs. Mills what the pills she has been given are. Grace assumes that Mrs. Mills is trying to drug or poison her, but Mrs. Mills answers that those are Grace's tablets for migraine. Another similar scene is when Mrs. Mills tells Mr. Tuttle and Lydia that the children will be easy to be dealt with, but Grace is more stubborn. This scene implies that the servants do have intentions that haven't been revealed yet and which Grace is likely to oppose, which corroborates that they are threatening. While Grace is absent from this scene, the conversation suggests that the servants are in opposition to the family, and the fact that the film is framed around the mother's perspective aligns the audience with her. In other words, because the audience's perspective is aligned with Grace, they are led to trust Grace's suspicions, and the servants are consequently viewed as ill-intentioned.

Studying horror films from the early to mid-twentieth century, Timothy Shary and Nancy McVittie notice a trend in these films to portray older women as scary. They argue that this stems from a growing anxiety about aging, which became more obvious in the post-war culture's focus on youth (Shary and McVittie 2016: 78). Both authors notice that the creation of horror films with specific focus on older women "renders the aging women at their core as monstrously 'othered' objects" (ibid.: 86). This otherness is exacerbated when combined with a sense of detachment from normal societal structures, like the nuclear family. In *The Others*, both the older servants, Mrs. Bertha Mills and Mr. Edmund Tuttle, are othered because they don't belong to the Stewart family. They are not familiar grandparents but unknown intruders, strongly contrasted against the young family. In the film, this sense of otherness is magnified by combining an emphasis on age with secrecy, heightened by the film's framing, reducing them to caricatures acting in very suspicious ways. Even though, Grace has no proof that the servants are responsible for what is happening in the house and the audience later learns that they are not intentionally causing any harm, their familiarity with the house, their sudden arrival, their secrecy, and the fact that in one of the scenes Mr. Tuttle appears possibly covering his own or Mrs. Mills' tombstone with dry leaves to hide it from view, emphasize the servant's role as unknown entities, and imply that they are the threat.

When it comes to disability, the strategy to transform it in alterity is similar to what happens to old age in films. Disability as a category is used in horror films to highlight bodily differences that appeal to existing societal assumptions about bodily impairments (Sutton 2017: 74). Writing about the concept of the norm, how its creation in the 1840s resulted in ideas about "abnormality" and in practices that created disability, Lennard J. Davis explains that the introduction of the idea of norm signifying "average" and "standard" created expectations that "the majority of the population must or should somehow be part of the norm" (Davis 2016: 3). The norm was informed by the work of statisticians (many of them eugenicists) such as Adolphe Quetelet, who applied mathematical notions to "the distribution of human features such as height and weight […] [and] […] formulat[ed] the concept of 'l'homme moyen' or 'the average man'" (ibid.: 3). By defining the norm through a series of mathematical equations and graphs, these statisticians created the circumstances that placed disabled bodies outside of what would be scientifically considered "normal" and made them, consequently, seen as deviant (ibid.: 3). This deviation from the norm is key to understanding why disabled bodies are portrayed as monstrous, that is, are othered. In *The Others*, while Lydia's speech disability is not immediately distinguishable, it gains a suspicious connotation as the film progresses: as Mrs. Bertha Mills and Mr. Edmund Tuttle become more suspicious due to their lack of surprise with the strange things happening in the house, Lydia's inability to speak can be read as an extension of their power over the household. She is often depicted being subservient to Mrs. Mills and Mr. Tuttle. Spectators are likely to believe that she has been coerced to keep mum about the intentions of the other two servants. In the end, when spectators realize the film had led us to believe that the three servants were dangerous when they were not, we discover that when Lydia was alive she didn't have a speech disability. Her speech disability developed when she realized that she had died.

In addition to Lydia's disability, Grace's likely mental illness also means she is disabled. Rosamarie Garland-Thomson corroborates this idea when she places disability and mental illness in the same "artificial category that encompasses congenital and acquired physical differences, mental illness [...] temporary or permanent injuries" (qtd. in Smith 2011: 4). Anne's accusations that her mother is mad, Grace's strange habits of locking doors behind her and the revelation at the end of the plot that Grace killed her children and herself are all indications that Grace may have a mental illness. If this is the case, why does it look like the servants may be posing a threat to the family? The revelation that Grace and her children are also ghosts exposes that Grace's perspective, which permeates and conducts most of the film, has always been unreliable. The unreliability of the characters enhances and magnifies ambiguities. Indeed, uncertainty is an important feature of the genre of ghost stories because it encompasses the struggle between relying on the material and rational world or on the supernatural (Bissell 2012: 40).

Writing about literature, scholar Julia Briggs understands that ghost stories are a category of the Gothic (2012: 177) and recognizes that they are "part of a wider reaction against the rationalism and [...] secularization of the Enlightenment, which [...] reflected in [...] new philosophies that set out to explore how knowledge was formulated in the mind and how the less conscious processes of the mind operated" (ibid. 2012: 179). A result of the opposition of rationalism is that, in ghost stories, rationality is questioned and the supernatural becomes as feasible as the rational (Long Hoeveler 2012: 23). This means that ghost stories represent a "challenge to the very notion of an agreed, verifiable reality [...] [and they present] a chance to [...] open up new questions about reality" (Brewster and Thuston 2018: 3). Therefore, ghost stories make space for people to explore their subjectivity and complexity. This often results in a scrutiny of what is in the realm of the familiar, not only because this tends to be intruded upon (Briggs 2012: 176) but because it may be a source of terror and fear.

In *The Others*, the ambiguities are not so much about the rational *versus* the supernatural world. Instead, they encompass different explanations of who or what is responsible for the chaos in the house and vary according to how much reliability characters are granted. Vera Nünning explains that narrative reliability enables crucial insights into how cultures operate. Nünning is interested in learning about narrative reliability beyond the realm of literature thus integrating it with other disciplines. From this comprehensive perspective, she asserts that "[j]udgements concerning unreliability [...] highlight the borderline between the normal and the deviant; they show those implicit norms, values, and personality theories that are part of the implicit cultural knowledge but rarely expressed in explicit terms" (Nünning 2015: 14). Her insights resonate with *The Others* especially when it comes to the portrayal of old age and disability and how untrustworthy the characters that are either old or disabled are. For instance, in the beginning of the film when Grace's habits enable her portrayal as quirky and her likely mental illness is not yet obvious, the monstrous, i.e. abject, depictions of old age and disability give some sense of stability to the film. When Grace starts asking questions about the servants to Mrs. Mills, but the latter gives Grace vague answers and soon goes about her work to evade more questions, the audience recognizes that there is something suspicious about Mrs. Mills. As long as spectators identify older and disabled people as the threats, the film offers us tools to navigate the complexity of the plot and ambiguities are obscured.

However, since the film is told from Grace's point of view, if Grace is mentally ill, the narrative that she is telling lacks a logic reliability so the audience may be left wondering what is really happening, which adds more instability and ambiguity to the narrative. Grace's possible mental illness connects her to the monstrous, that is, the abject, and, more importantly, it suggests that she may not be a reliable narrator. In addition to discovering who or what the threat is, Grace's possible lack of reliability complicates the plot further because there seems to be nothing about the film that is normal, logical or coherent. As a result, spectators are likely to question if the servants actually pose a threat especially as Mrs. Mills often seems to be more understanding and level-headed towards Anne than her own mother. While scenes that show servants discussing upcoming changes amongst themselves continue to corroborate Grace's distrust of the servants, spectators are likely to consider if there are answers to the mysteries of the house that we haven't accessed yet.

In an examination about the role of novels in the creation of disability, Davis argues that novels were used to impose normative structures and enforce ideas about normalcy (2016: 9). Similarly, films, and especially horror films with ideas of what or who can be monstrous, also function corroborating notions of normalcy and average. Since it is unclear if Grace is really going mad or if the servants are plotting against the family and haunting the house, it is difficult for spectators to make sense of what is going on or where to locate the expected normalcy that Davis recognizes in narratives. Moreover, spectators are not likely to believe the children because their age suggests that both Anne and Nicholas are unreliable. Lastly, Anne claims that she sees ghosts, a statement that appears to defy logic and makes her untrustworthy for most of the film.

The lack of clear logic and the uncertainties of the plot are materialized in the constant fog that surrounds the haunted house the Stewart family and the servants inhabit. As demonstrated by the scene in which Grace decides to venture outside of the house to look for her husband and then returns home because she fears getting lost in the fog, the plot of the film leaves important information out thus making spectators feel as if we are also lost in the fog. The ghosts and the fog also add to the horror/ghost story atmosphere and indicate that the plot is set in a haunted house. Surrounded by fog, the house is almost like a character itself, especially as its inhabitants hear the piano in the empty, dark room being played and it seems like the house has a life of its own. In *Danse Macabre*, Stephen King explains that a "haunted house" or a "bad place" (as he calls any spaces that elicit fear) is a "house with unsavory history" (qtd. in Freeman 2018: 328). The many uncertainties in the plot of the film hint at the possibility of a house with an unsavory history.

The film reveals its plot twist in two stages, first revealing that the servants are ghosts, then dismantling the narrative reliability in the séance scene where Grace, Anne and Nicholas discover that they are also dead and ghosts. The fact that they are ghosts and the manner in which they died links back to the idea of a house with an unsavory history. In this case, instead of overlooking death, which is what Briefel suggests they are doing (96) by being unable to acknowledge their status as deceased, Grace and the children are repressing their knowledge of being dead. In *Ghostly Matters: Haunting and the Sociological Imagination*, Avery F. Gordon explains that ghosts have a real connection to the material world because "[t]he whole essence [...] of a ghost is that it has a real presence and demands its due, your attention" (2008: xvi). In the film, the ghost servants and the living inhabitants of the house that are initially perceived as ghosts do receive the attention of the Stewart family and, consequently, of the spectators. However, later in the film we learn that this is a mere distraction from what has really happened, that is, Grace's suffocating her children before killing herself. When it comes to the narrative, this is also a distraction that functions to not give the plot away even if throughout the film, the audience is given hints about what has happened to the family, such as when Grace walks into a room whose furniture is covered in white sheets that look like ghosts. Their fate lingers in the film, but it takes time for them to acknowledge it.

Freud's uncanny is useful to understand why, beyond their old age and disability, the servants are scary to the family. According to Freud, "the uncanny [*unheimlich*] is something that is secretly familiar [*heimlich-heimisch*] which has undergone repression and has returned from it" (2001: 245). The act of repression is never fully successful because the uncanny tends to recur producing fear (ibid.: 241). To the Stewart family, the servants are scary because their status as dead people is eerily familiar, that is, somehow known. The servants evoke the uncanny because they represent what Grace and the children have become but are trying to repress and, consequently, the family literally feels haunted by their counterparts. As the plot unfolds, Graces feels increasingly restless because it becomes more and more difficult to repress her knowledge and memories. One pivotal moment in the film is when her husband returns from the war in a state of shell shock and soon after leaves. This is when chaos ensues. The curtains covering the windows are completely removed and light starts to get in. The light illuminating the house functions as a metaphor showing that Grace is getting closer to the truth about what happened to the children and her, which she has repressed. The haunted house is often read as a "metaphor for the mysteries of the mind" (Bissell 2012: 45), so the light getting in brings clarity to those that have been in the dark. An example of this clarity is when Grace's memories return in the séance scene resolving the complexity of the plot and matters of unreliability. In this scene, Anne whispers to the Old Lady, an old woman with cataracts, that her mother suffocated her and her brother with a pillow and then shot herself. Even though this plot twist seems to undo the connection of old age and disability to monstrosity because it becomes obvious that the servants are not the menace, the old woman's ability to communicate with the afterlife still displays a connection with the abject because of the trespassing of borders and the proximity to the dead.

A previous scene had already shown the Old Lady as monstrous. This scene is one of the most disturbing in the film and it reinforces ageist and ableist stereotypes. It shows Anne being possessed by the old woman. When Grace gets closer, instead of Anne, she sees an old woman with cataracts that speaks with Anne's voice. Moreover, where we expect Anne to be sitting, we see an old hand maneuvering a puppet and the Old Lady is wearing Anne's First Communion dress. Grace is so frightened that she tries to suffocate the old woman, who then transforms into Anne. This scene elicits fear because of the stark contrast between Anne's young age and the old woman that is produced when Grace looks closely and doesn't see Anne. When Grace and the spectators discover that this is, in fact, an old woman, this gives everyone a scare. With so much information being left out of the plot, this scene makes the spectator question if Anne had been an old woman all along. If this hypothesis is true, the film embodies the horror and the grotesque because of characters' possible inability to acknowledge the passing of time (Chivers 2011: 45). However, the old woman soon transforms into Anne and the audience has to rule this hypothesis out. This scene isn't scary because the characters are unable to perceive the passing of time and then suddenly encounter irrefutable proof of aging. Instead, more than showing the old body as abject this scene magnifies fear by portraying the old woman as if *she* hadn't acknowledged the passing of time and hadn't realized that she is not a child anymore. But, in the end, this is not true either as the old woman doesn't seem to be unable to recognize her own age.

The truth is that Grace and her children were the ones who were unable to acknowledge the passing of time because they had been living in a fixed time frame. They weren't trying to forgo aging. Instead, their fate was the result of the experiences the family was subjected to: the Nazi occupation of the island of Jersey and Grace hearing that her husband had probably died in France, where he was deployed. That is, the family's inability to acknowledge the passing of time has more to do with grief and trauma than an attempt to avoid aging. This realization about the Stewart family has, as an effect, a normalization of what had previously been portrayed as abnormal and monstrous. We then gather that the war and its effects on the family were so horrific and devastating that, in comparison, the servants and the old woman lose some of their status as abjection, while Grace and her children become more abject because of their status as dead people and their shocking death.

When the tensions resolve and spectators have all the pieces of the puzzle to make sense of this complex plot, we understand that the ambiguities that trespass boundaries and make the self feel repugnant or fear-inducing don't have to be resolved. They don't have to be separated by rigid boundaries that protect the self as Kristeva suggests. In the end of the film, the dead and living must coexist. Similarly, the Stewart family must learn to live together with Mrs. Mill, Mr. Tuttle and Lydia. Of interest here is how this idea makes the boundaries between old and young, able and disabled more porous. Instead of seeing old age and disability as undesired features that one cannot get rid of, the characters learn to embody contradicting, inherent features with no consequence to their reliability. The knowledge of the contradictory embodiments that the different characters comprise doesn't make them any less sinister than they were before, but perhaps more human and even relatable because their experiences offer spectators the opportunity to explore our own complexities, and perhaps even our own biases against older and disabled people.

Acknowledgments

To Jessica Anne Carter for proofreading, editing and giving advice; to João Paulo Guimarães for the soft deadlines; to Isobel Jellema for reading previous versions of this chapter; to Dr. Amy J. Vosper for recommending important literature on horror film and to Lyzee Ninham for the encouragement, a big thank you!

Author Bio

Mariana Castelli-Rosa is a PhD candidate (Cultural Studies) at Trent University, Canada. She has two MAs (English Studies from the University of Heidelberg, Germany and Public Texts from Trent University, Canada) and a BA in English and Portuguese and a Teaching Degree from the University of São Paulo, Brazil. Her areas of interest are Canadian and Indigenous literatures, cultural understandings and images of aging; translation and tensions in intercultural encounters; interactions between countries and individuals from the Global South and so-called developed countries and how these may shape identity; trauma, popular culture, identity, gender. She currently works as a Teaching Assistant and Marker at the Department of Gender and Social Justice at Trent University. She also works as a Research Assistant editing and annotating through coding the journal that Canadian poet PK Page wrote during her time in Brazil and Robertson Davies' Massey College diaries. She is an aspiring academic and translator and her doctoral research is on the experience of aging in Indigenous communities in Canada through the analysis of works of life writing and novels.

Works Cited

Amenábar, Alejandro. The Others. 2001.
Benshoff, Harry M. (2017): "Preface." In: Harry M. Benshoff (ed.), A Companion to the Horror Film, Chichester: Wiley Blackwell. \
Bissell, Sarah (2018): "The Ghost Story and Science." In: Scott Brewster/ Luke Thurston (eds.), The Routledge Handbook to the Ghost Story, New York and London: Routledge.

Brewster, Scott/Thurston, Luke (2018): "Introduction." In: Scott Brewster/Luke Thurston (eds.), The Routledge Handbook to the Ghost Story, New York and London: Routledge.

Briefel, Aviva (2009): "What Some Ghosts Don't Know: Spectral Incognizance and the Horror Film." In: Narrative 17/1, pp. 95–110.

Briggs, Julia (2012): "The Ghost Story." In: David Punter (ed.), A New Company to the Gothic, Oxford: Blackwell.

Chivers, Sally (2011): The Silvering Screen: Old Age and Disability in Cinema, Toronto: University of Toronto Press.

Chivers, Sally/Markotić, Nicole (2010): "Introduction." In: Sally Chivers/Nicole Markotić (eds.), The Problem Body: Projecting Disability in Film, Columbus: Ohio State University Press.

Davis, Lennard J. (2016): "Introduction: Disability, Normality and Power" In: Lennard J. Davis (ed.), The Disability Studies Reader, New York: Routledge.

Freeman, Nick (2018): "Haunted Houses." In: Scott Brewster/Luke Thurston (eds.), The Routledge Handbook to the Ghost Story, New York and London: Routledge.

Freud, Sigmund (2001): "The Uncanny." In: Alix Strachley/Alan Tyson (eds.), The Standard Edition of the Complete Psychological Works of Sigmund Freud. Vol. 17, An Infantile Neurosis; and Other Works: (1917–1919), London: The Hogarth Press and The Institute of Psychoanalysis.

Gordon, Avery F. (2008): Ghostly Matters: Haunting and the Sociological Imagination, Minneapolis: University of Minnesota Press.

Kristeva, Julia (1982): Powers of Horror: An Essay on Abjection, New York: Columbia University Press.

Long Hoeveler, Diane (2018): "Gothic and Romantic Ghosts in Novels, Dramas, and the Chapbook." In: Scott Brewster/Luke Thurston (eds.), The Routledge Handbook to the Ghost Story, New York and London: Routledge.

Nünning, Vera (2015): "Conceptualising (Un)reliable Narration and (Un)trustworthiness" In: Vera Nünning (ed.), Unreliable Narration and Trustworthiness: Intermedial and Interdisciplinary Perspectives, Berlin/Munich/Boston: De Gruyter.

Shary, Timothy/McVittie, Nancy (2016): Fade to Gray: Aging in American Cinema, Austin: University of Texas Press.

Smajić, Srdjan (2010): Ghost-Seers, Detectives, and Spiritualists: Theories of Vision in Victorian Literature and Science, Cambridge: Cambridge University Press.

Smith, Angela M. (2011): Hideous Progeny: Disability, Eugenics, and Classic Horror Cinema, New York: Columbia University Press.

Sutton, Travis (2017): "Avenging the Body: Disability in the Horror Film." In: Harry M. Benshoff (ed.), A Companion to the Horror Film, Chichester: Wiley Blackwell.

Worland, Rick (2007): The Horror Film: An Introduction, Oxford: Blackwell Publishing.

Fears of Old Age, Cultural Representations of Elders and Narrative Twists of Aging in Four Horror Episodes of the *Twilight Zone*

Marta Miquel-Baldellou[1]

Introduction

In his comprehensive essay on horror fiction, *Danse Macabre*, which comprises the analysis of the most relevant novels and films in the history of the genre, American writer Stephen King highlights the importance of Rod Serling's pioneering original television series *The Twilight Zone* (2000, 260). Authors who shifted comfortably from novels to screenwriting contributed many scripts to the series, as is the case with Charles Beaumont, George Clayton Johnson and, particularly, Richard Matheson, whom King has credited as one of the basic inspirations for his career (Nolan 2009, 10). As King further claims, *The Twilight Zone* was rooted in "solid concepts which form a vital link between the old pulp fiction predating the fifties and the new literature of horror," while he cherished that each episode introduced "ordinary people in extraordinary situations, people who had somehow turned sideways and slipped through a crack in reality" (2000: 276), which is one of the main reasons for which King has also been praised as one of the masters of contemporary horror fiction.

The Twilight Zone was an American anthology series which ran on CBS for five seasons, from 1959 to 1964, attracting popular and critical

---

[1] University of Lleida.

acclaim on equal terms. Pertaining to genres ranging from horror and fantasy to science fiction, *The Twilight Zone* presented a series of episodes, which were independent from each other, in terms of plot, characters, setting, and script, while the technical staff, comprising cast, directors, and screenwriters, also differed in each episode. According to William Boddy, though, all the episodes displayed narratological continuities (1984: 107), such as Rod Serling's voice-over, whose omniscient comments introduced and brought each piece to an end, and its narrative structure, which involved a short presentation of the situation that set the plot in motion, the introduction of the bizarre before a pause for commercials, and a surprising twist which implied a change in perspective and provided a final coda which was evocative of a modern moral fable.

An analysis of the episodes in the original five seasons of the series exposes that aging reveals itself as a recurring theme that is discussed from manifold perspectives. In its own plural dimensions, aging arises as a particularly appropriate and malleable theme from a narratological point of view to be approached through the genres of horror, fantasy, and science fiction. In the different seasons of the series, a variety of subjects inextricably related to the discourses of aging are tackled, such as magical potions that provide eternal youth, the blurring edges of life stages, the almighty power that elders may exert over the youth, scientific breakthroughs that extend life beyond its natural limits, intergenerational conflicts, and the fizzy boundaries that separate life from death (Miquel-Baldellou 2016: 113). In many of these narratives that explicitly address aging, the portrayal of old characters often evokes cultural images traditionally associated with the aged, which Herbert Covey (1991) identifies as patriarchs endowed with some spiritual dimension that transcends death, personifications of the sage or the witch derived from popular folklore, misers exerting a tight economic control as legacy of traditional family structures, sentimentalized elders in their grandparental roles, and aged individuals who defy the established cultural dictates of aging and are portrayed as ludicrous and grotesque.

Anxieties and fears related to aging and the aged are discussed in different episodes of *The Twilight Zone* that are categorized within the horror genre. Even if mostly set in American middle-class suburbs at the end of the fifties and early sixties, the horror narratives of *The Twilight Zone* comply with most of the tenets pertaining to the Gothic tradition that critics like David Stevens point out, such as the fascination with the past, the juxtaposition of reality and the supernatural, the exploration of the unconscious, the exploitation of the sinister and the macabre, the alienation of domestic scenarios, and the structural disposition of plots within plots which favors subjectivity and a shift of perspective (2010: 46). The ambiguous nature that characterizes horror, together with the recurrent narratological structure of reversing the initial situation that typifies each of the narratives, paves the way for the ambivalent portrayal of old age that is fostered in *The Twilight Zone*. According to Cynthia J. Miller and A. Bowdoin van Riper, contemporary filmic narratives that deal with aging mostly reflect "ambivalent attitudes toward growing old" (2019, 1), as elders are characterized in the roles of either victims or villains, and the fears of aging that are explored range from the dread of aging badly through dependence and illness to the fearful fantasies of abject bodies returning back to life to haunt their younger counterparts. Many decades prior to the release of contemporary horror films that explore the anxieties of aging and present an ambiguous portrait of old age, *The Twilight Zone* produced a series of horror narratives which explicitly addressed old age and called into question culturally assumed notions about aging.

An analysis of four horror narratives in *The Twilight Zone* which explore different fears related to the discourses of aging will serve the purpose of identifying how cultural perceptions of old age are constructed and disrupted, thus providing an eminently ambiguous portrayal of aging, and evoking and subverting the ways the aged and the youth are represented in popular culture. The first narrative that will be addressed in this essay is "Night Call" for which Richard Matheson wrote its screen narrative based on his own short story featuring Elva Keene, an aged woman who starts receiving some mysterious phone calls in the middle of the night. In "Spur of the Moment," with a script also written by Matheson, a young girl, Anne Henderson, flees in terror as she is chased by a terrifying aging woman dressed in black. "Nothing in the Dark," written by George Clayton Johnson, portrays the last days of Wanda Dunn, an aged woman who encloses herself at home out of fear with the hope of escaping death in old age. Finally, with a script written by Charles Beaumont and William Idelson, "Long Distance Call" tells the story of five-year-old boy Billy Bayles who speaks to his late grandmother on the toy phone she gave him as a present for his birthday. By means of narratological elements pertaining to the horror genre, but also through the underlying structure of the series that plays with the audience's expectations and resorts to unexpected final twists of the plot, these four narratives evoke, as well as subvert, popular beliefs of aging and the contrasting representation of youth and old age. This essay aims at analysing the ways in which these four horror narratives evoke cultural assumptions which associate old age with determinate values only to disrupt them and provide an ambivalent and twilight portrayal which fosters critical thinking and the revision of socially-accepted representations of elders and old age.

Beware of the Victimized Loner: Fears of Aging Badly in "Night Call"

"Night Call" portrays the apparently uneventful life of Miss Elva Keene, an older woman who lives alone in a rural community in Maine, when, all of a sudden, she starts receiving disturbing phone calls at night. Based on Richard Matheson's short-story "Long Distance Call," which was originally published with the title "Sorry, Right Number," and adapted to the screen also with a script written by Matheson, "Night Call" consists of tale of horror which addresses the fears of aging, and in particular, as Cynthia Miller and A. Bowdoin van Riper would say, the "fears of aging badly" as a result of envisioning old age as a degenerative process and of presenting the elderly as struggling with marginalization and victimization (2019: 1). At the beginning of both the original story and its screen adaptation, Elva's aging traits are constantly highlighted, thus contributing to constructing a portrayal of old age mostly characterized by dependence and physical decline.

In Matheson's short story, attention is drawn to Elva's difficulty in carrying out her daily routines which often bring her close to the point of fatigue and exhaustion,
stating that, "her thin hand faltered in the darkness," "her infirm back ached from effort of sitting," and "she forced out a weary breath" (2008: 253), while "she couldn't stretch far enough and crippled legs prevented her from rising" (2008: 255). An early passage in the narrative also informs about the monotony of her existence, as it is claimed that "life for Miss Keene was the sorry pattern of lying flat or being propped on pillows, reading books which Nurse Phillips brought from the town library, getting nourishment, rest, medication, listening to her tiny radio-and waiting, *waiting* for something different to happen" (254). In its screen adaptation, the aging traits of the character are also emphasized through close-up shots of actress Gladys Cooper, which highlight her white hair and the lines on her face. Her clothes also contribute significantly to stressing old age, as Elva often wraps her shoulders with a cardigan or a woolen scarf. Props like a wheelchair, pill bottles, and a glass of milk on her bedside table, together with the ever presence of Nurse Margaret Phillips, are constant reminders of Elva's permanent convalescence and expose that she is in need of constant care. Elva's portrayal as an older woman complies with Sally Chivers's premises about commonly held assumptions that associate the aged body with disability (2013: 8), which contribute to envisioning old age as mostly linked with invalidism, dependence, inactivity, and loneliness. These dramaturgical props, which are often linked with old age in popular culture, also reveal the role that cultural discourses play to categorise individuals as aged (Gullette 2004: 12), hence exposing old age as an eminently cultural construct.

Nonetheless, Elva's tedious existence is suddenly brought to a halt when she begins to receive some mysterious phone calls in the middle of the night. The phone calls pave the way for the fantastic to make its appearance in the safe haven of Elva's domesticity. As the narrative unfolds, many elements indicative of classic gothic trappings are displayed cinematically, while, in narratological terms, the narrative remains entirely focalized on Elva's as a character. The cinematic style of the episode is allusive of its director, Jacques Tourneur, the French film director, who was particularly influenced by German expressionism and the films of directors such as F.W. Murnau, Fritz Lang, and Robert Wiene, and whose cinematic techniques gave precedence to subjective perspectives and the distortion of reality for the sake of emotional effect. By means of extreme close-up shots of Elva, the narrative remains focalized on her perception of reality, while an opening chiaroscuro scene, with looming shadows superimposing on Elva, highlights an impending sense of danger which signals Elva as its besieged victim, and contributes to increasing the audience's feelings of fear and anxiety.

Among the distinctive elements of the Gothic tradition that this narrative displays, the initial sequence portrays an isolated house and resorts to darkness, stormy weather, and particularly, the sound of thunder as the response to Elva's answering the phone in the middle of the night. The mysterious origins of these calls underpin Tzvetan Todorov's disjunctive between "the marvelous" and "the uncanny" as different ways to account for the fantastic (1975: 41–42). The sound of thunder as a response to Elva's queries seems to indicate a sign from the transcendence, thus hinting at "the marvelous," rather than "the uncanny," as the basis of this puzzle. Nevertheless, the explanation for these enigmatic calls may still simply lie in the phone's bad connection in such stormy weather, which would make room for the "uncanny," on account of which apparently supernatural phenomena turn out to have a rational explanation. This second hypothesis seems more feasible when the following morning Elva calls the phone company to inquire about these mysterious calls and the young operator, Miss Finch, informs her that the phone line has probably been damaged during the storm.

The two young women that Elva interacts with on a daily basis, Miss Finch and Nurse Phillips, often bring to the fore prevalent social prejudices against the elderly. In Matheson's story, it is stated that "Miss Finch thought she [Elva] was a nervous old woman falling prey to imagination" (2008: 259), and when Elva tells her nurse that she thinks the person responsible for those mysterious calls is a man, Nurse Phillips retorts, "you don't have to talk to him. Just hang up. Is that so hard to do?" (2008: 261). Nurse Phillips's words subtly unveil social prescriptions that disapprove of sexuality in old age. As Covey argues, the notion of romantic love has often been regarded as age inappropriate for older people (1991: 112), particularly for women, given the conventional assumption that sexual desire ends with menopause. Taking Elva's statements about a whispering male voice calling her in the middle of the night as the result of an aged woman's romantic flights of fancy, both Nurse Phillips and Miss Finch dismiss Elva's account of the facts as eccentric and even ridiculous in a portrait not entirely unlike that of Miss Havisham. Like Dickens's ghostly character in *Great Expectations*, Miss Elva Keene often appears as dressed in white, she hardly ever leaves home and, given the constant appellation to her marital status at her age, she is considered a "spinster" concealing a mysterious and tragic love story which took place in her youth.

This succession of calls from a mysterious male voice has an ambivalent effect on Elva and her attitude toward them. At first, she feels both pestered and terrified upon hearing the frightening moans and almost inarticulate speech from a stranger's male voice. Nonetheless, in a subtle, and even ironic, way, these calls seem to give her a purpose and she even grows restless upon expecting them in the evening, as if waiting for somebody she could eventually talk to and finally bring her loneliness to an end. This transformation shows in Elva's appearance, which gradually undergoes a symbolic process of rejuvenation that becomes perceptible through her choice of clothes and hairstyle. This self-induced change on Elva's looks calls to mind Anne Basting's premise about the "performative nature of aging" (1998: 4), Margaret Gullette's precepts about acting younger or older (2004: 168) regardless of one's chronological age, and Kathleen Woodward's notion about aging being performed in correlation with gender (2006: 165). However, according to Barbara Walker, displays of sexual allure on behalf of postmenopausal women have been considered "a moral evil" (1985: 90) and aging women who evince sexual interest have often been judged as grotesque and even socially threatening. As a result of these precepts, a subsequent moral retribution finds its way when Elva's positive prospects take a turn for the worse. Miss Finch, the telephone operator, calls Elva to tell her that there is no way any man could have called her on the previous nights because the repairmen have traced the wire which fell down during the storm and caused the phone line massive damage, ultimately finding out that the wire is lying on the outskirts of town and, in fact, in one of the graves of the cemetery.

After this shocking revelation, the plot comes to an end in a differing way in Matheson's original story and its screen adaptation. In the short story, after Elva is informed that the calls have been traced as coming from the graveyard, she receives a highly disturbing final call in which the speaker tells her, "Hello, Miss Elva. I'll be right over" (265). This unsettling statement complies with what King terms as 'terror' as opposed to 'horror,' since it is rather "what the mind imagines [rather than what the eye sees] what makes a story a quintessential tale of terror" worthy of its name (2000: 36). At a literal level, as an example of 'horror,' the reader may picture a walking corpse creeping on its way to Elva's home, which would be somehow evocative of the end in W.W. Jacobs's story "The Paw," but, at a more metaphorical level, as indicative of 'terror,' the conclusion in the original story rather points at Death finally knocking on Elva's door, which brings to the fore the fear of death in old age, in the still of the night, when Elva is alone and helpless in her bed.

In contrast, the ending of Matheson's screen adaptation rather emphasizes notions of sin, guilt, and retribution which comply with the narratological features of *The Twilight Zone* and endow this horror story with some of the components of a moral fable. As Matheson explains in relation to the recurrent narratological structure of the series, "structurally, we all did the same thing, which was to start out with a little teaser that gets the viewer interested, and then have a little suspense item at the end of the first act, and then resolving it through the script, through the story, and then finishing it with a surprise ending, or at the very least, some kind of ironic observation regarding the story" (Stanyard 2007: 162). The surprising turn that the plot takes in Matheson's screen adaptation seems grounded in a passage from the original story in which it is unveiled that, while lying in bed and unable to sleep, Elva feels compelled to "turn the faucet in her brain and keep unwanted thoughts from dripping" (2008: 254), which subtly underscores Elva's latent sense of guilt for some unknown reason. In the screen adaptation, Nurse Phillips finally takes Elva to the cemetery, where the older woman realises that the damaged telephone wire is lying within the grave of her late fiancé, Brian, who died in a car accident for which she was to blame. Elva tells Nurse Phillips that she was very dominating and Brian always did what she said, so she insisted on driving, causing an accident which killed Brian and rendered her unable to walk for life. According to Carl Plantinga, this conclusion could be categorized as a surprising turn whereby "the ending is surprising for the spectator, but not so for the character" (45), since, by means of a twist of the plot, the viewer's initial thoughts on Elva shift significantly, as she moves from being initially victimized to being eventually vilified. Upon knowing that the mysterious caller is her late fiancé, Elva feels relieved that she will finally have someone to talk to. Nonetheless, as a result of cosmic irony, when he calls her that night, he refuses to talk to her on the grounds that, on the previous call, she told him to leave her alone, and so he retorts this is what he will do since he always does what she says. "Night Call" thus turns into what Noël Carroll considers a "tale of dread" (1990: 42), insofar as it involves some sort of cosmic moral justice and it is hinted that Elva is eventually punished for her past sins. This ironic, but tragic, turn of prospects, paves the way for an open ending, which can be interpreted as either Brian's ghost finally taking revenge on his fiancée, or simply Elva's ghost of conscience punishing herself as a result of unsurmountable guilt in her old age.

From a narratological perspective, this episode displays a circular structure which enacts the transformation of Elva's portrayal as an aged woman. The initial close-up shot of Elva's wheelchair categorizes her as a victim, and depicts Elva as helpless and dependent. Conversely, at its close, given the change of prospects, Elva's wheelchair is a reminder of the accident for which she is held responsible for her fiancé's death and her own disabled condition. Since Elva is gradually portrayed from victim to villain, her depiction as an older woman offers an ambivalent portrayal of old age, as she is subjected to a process of victimization first only to be disclosed that she is to blame and is, in fact, punished eventually as a result of poetic justice. The ending of Matheson's screen adaptation is somehow evocative of Robert Aldrich's film *What Ever Happened to Baby Jane?* which was released only two years before "Night Call" was broadcast on television. Baby Jane is first portrayed as a sadistic and alcoholic older woman, apparently guilty of causing the accident which incapacitated her sister Blanche. Nonetheless, it is later on revealed that, in spite of her innocent appearance, Blanche is accountable for her own disabled condition, as so is Elva in Matheson's script. In comparison with Matheson's original short story, whereby the reader imagines a walking corpse creeping off to Elva's place or, metaphorically, the figure of Death finally knocking on Elva's door, his screen adaptation rather suggests that there may be something more terrifying than death for Elva, which is loneliness in old age and, particularly, the burden of haunting memories as a result of an unyielding sense of guilt.

Afraid of the Aging Rider: the Dread of Recognizing Oneself as Old in "Spur of the Moment"

With a script also written by Matheson and under the direction of Elliot Silverstein, "Spur of the Moment" was originally broadcast only a couple of weeks after "Night Call." From its onset, this film acquires the aura of an intriguing fairy tale. In the first scene, a young woman, Anne Henderson, who is to be married to a wealthy man, Robert, against her will, because she is actually in love with David, whom her parents strongly disapprove of, leaves from an elegant country house to ride her horse when, all of a sudden, she begins to be chased violently by a mysterious aging woman, who is also on horseback, but is all dressed in black. Given the resemblance of this story with an eerie fairy tale, the image of the aging woman in black is highly evocative of the folktale character of the witch. According to Covey, older women have ancestrally been associated with witchcraft, as the iconic representation of the witch in popular folklore corresponds with that of "an old woman, dressed in black, and riding a broomstick" (71), thus resembling the portrayal of this aging woman in black that haunts Anne.

This vociferous and wild older woman is described in Rod Serling's voice-over teaser at the beginning of the episode as "a strange, nightmarish figure of a woman in black, who has appeared as if from nowhere and now, at driving gallop, chases the terrified girl across the countryside, as if she means to ride her down and kill her." As an aging woman yelling at her victim, she becomes a source of the abject, which Julia Kristeva defines as the feeling that one experiences upon being confronted by a breakdown in the distinction between what is self and what is other. To use Kristeva's terms, "the abject appears in order to uphold 'I' within the Other," insofar as "it takes the ego back to its source on the abominable limits from which, in order to be, the ego has broken away" (1982: 15). Being both on horseback and enacting the same scene recurrently, it is suggested that the alienating figure of the aging woman in black may actually be closer to young Anne that she may even dare to think.

As the story unfolds and the terrified young girl goes back home to tell her parents and fiancé about the frightening aging woman who has been chasing her, in a mirrored scene, the aging woman also goes back home, to the same country house, where she unveils to her remarkably aged mother the following revelation:

> You know who I saw today? I saw a ghost, Mother. My own. Intriguing, isn't it? To be haunted by one's own self. Positively intriguing. I'm talking about ghosts, Mother. Phantoms, visitations, reminders from the past and the future. I went out riding today, out where I usually go, beyond the meadow. I was on the ridge, and I saw this young girl ride toward me. Me, Mother, as I looked at eighteen.

It is thus disclosed that the aging woman in black who chases young Anne at the beginning of the episode is, in fact, her older self. As she puts forward this revelation, she is standing as an older woman in front of a portrait of herself which was painted when she was young, so that her younger and older selves are visually juxtaposed in order to substantiate her explanation of the facts. This overlapping, and also disentanglement, of youth and old age bring about the shift in the focalization of the narrative voice that is to follow, which draws attention to the alternation of identities between these two symbolic doubles, thus questioning which of them stands for the source of the abject. For the young woman who looks terrified when the episode starts, the older woman becomes the Other, whereas for the older woman whose identity is revealed half through the narrative, it is her younger self whom she identifies as the source of her nightmarish existence and who urges her to chase her and warn her not to marry the wrong man.

The plot of this episode is narratologically structured along the combination of two different timeframes impinging on one another and, in this respect, Stewart Stanyard categorizes this narrative among those addressing the theme of time travel in the series (2007: 50). The implicit encroachment of the past into the present and the present back to the past explores the cyclical quality of life stages, thus suggesting that youth and old age are inherently related to one another instead of far removed from each other by means of the establishment of time boundaries. This interpretation is reinforced through dramaturgical props which either conceal or emphasize old age, thus underscoring the constructed quality of aging and, by extension, of the passage of time. The same actress, Diana Hyland, plays both roles as younger and older Anne, which lays bare how aging is visually counterfeited on the screen through resorting to what Margaret Gullette has referred to as "age effects" (2004: 171) both in terms of make-up and acting techniques. Along Hyland's performance of Anne's older self in her decadent mansion, close-up shots of her face stress her lines and wrinkles, incipient white hair, and the dark circles under her eyes. Her gestures denote lack of energy and passivity, which match her haggard look and distinctive nonchalance. Conversely, though, Anne's older self is also characterized as enraged and vigorous in the presence of her younger self, who, in contrast, feels overwhelmed and weakened by the haunting aging woman who rides in her pursuit.

As the narrative focalizes on Anne's older self, initial suspicions about the aging woman being a witch are left behind in favor of perceiving this older woman as a resolute fairy who wishes to warn her younger and more ingenuous self. Ironically, though, Anne's younger self is reluctant to listen to the aging woman's good advice given her prejudice and fear of the older woman, which leads her to categorize her as a devilish creature whose sole purpose must be that of killing her. Insofar as, at the beginning of the episode, Anne is about to marry Robert to please her family, it is assumed that Anne's haunting older self is visiting her younger self in order to warn her not to marry for money, but for love. Nonetheless, it is actually the other way round, since Anne's older self intends to prevent her younger self from making a last-minute mistake, as it is revealed that, on the spur of the moment, Anne finally decided to leave her wealthy fiancé Robert and marry David instead, whom she perceived to be her true love at the time.

As a coda to this gloomy and moralizing fairy tale, it is suggested that what is really frightening is not the older woman and her apparent terrifying demeanor, but rather the younger self's preconceptions about her, especially taking into consideration that, as it is unveiled through a display of dramatic irony, this older woman is, in fact, Anne herself. Her younger self's misjudgment is thus evocative of Simone de Beauvoir's claim about our inability to recognize ourselves as old, since, as Kathleen Woodward claims, Beauvoir notices that "we are not old; it is the other, the stranger within us who is old," ultimately arguing that old age belongs to the category of "the unrealizables" (Woodward 1983: 55). As Woodward further notices, "the recognition of our own old age comes to us from the Other" so that "we ultimately are forced to acknowledge the point of view of the Other that has, as it were, installed itself in our body" (1983: 56). Hence, the source of the abject truly lies in Anne's inability to identify herself as old, her alienated perception of herself, and her dread of recognizing herself as aged from the other's perspective.

The narratological disposition of Matheson's script plays with the audience's expectations and the cultural values associated with youth and old age only to subvert them and challenge them subsequently. As happens with "Night Call," "Spur of the Moment" presents a circular structure that refers back to its initial scene and introduces a significant change in perspective. When the story comes to a close, the narrative is not focalized on Anne's younger self, but on her older self, which is no longer perceived as alienating. Upon having met Anne's older self, it is rather her younger self which the spectator holds in contempt as a result of her poor judgement, while her older self finally turns out to be an agent of good will coming to Anne's rescue in spite of her apparently frightening looks.

The initial portrayal of old age in this episode is rooted in folklore representations of aging women as witches, who were ostracized as a result of their presumed latent power and became ancestral embodiments of social disquiet. The depiction of this aging woman as a source of the abject underpins social prejudices of aged women envisioned as keepers of wisdom and ancestral knowledge. This narrative also explores the fears of aging related to feelings of regret for the mistakes made in youth which can no longer be redeemed and whose effects still prevail in old age. Above all, though, "Spur of the Moment" addresses the psychological implications of not recognizing oneself as old, but rather identifying the aging double as the haunting incarnation of our deepest fears and anxieties.

Let the Young One In: Exploring the Horror of Death in "Nothing in the Dark"

The representation of old age offered in "Nothing in the Dark" is initially rooted in conventional representations of the aged as associated with isolation, poverty, physical fragility, mental instability, and nostalgia for the past. In particular, in his thematic classification of *The Twilight Zone*, Stanyard refers to "Nothing in the Dark" as one of the episodes exploring the experience of dying (2007: 35), insofar as it tackles the will to hold on stubbornly to life in old age as a result of an extreme fear of death. With a script written by George Clayton Johnson, the symbolic and transcendent content of "Nothing in the Dark" complies with its author's beliefs of what fantasy should involve, since "it must be about the human condition" (Zicree 1992: 166). As a moral parable, this episode arises as an allegory which metaphorically exemplifies the physical and spiritual movement from darkness into the light, as the female protagonist gains insight into the experience of dying and, accordingly, her perception of the ways to approach the last stage of existence and even death undergoes an important change.

In "Nothing in the Dark," Wanda Dunn, played by Gladys Copper, locks herself up in her basement apartment during the remaining years of her old age with the determination of escaping Death. To that purpose, she lives in utter isolation and refuses to open the door to any unexpected guest in case Death may finally make its entry into her permanently sheltered, but also, constraining existence. In an initial scene, Wanda is first shown lying in her disheveled bed, protected with chairs carefully propped against its sides in order to avoid any fall that may bring her closer to the much dreaded and constantly projected end of her life. Her obsessive concern to protect herself from the world outside is exposed by means of frames that emphasize her perpetual enclosure, such as when her face shows behind the bars of her shielding, but imposing, headboard. Wanda thus seems unaware that, owing to her wish to overcome any predictable danger that may threaten her already wavering existence, she may actually be condemning herself to a virtual life-in-death. An initial close-up of Wanda's face brings attention to her white hair and her wrinkled features, as she lies helplessly in her bed. Despite being apparently asleep, her face still betrays an acute sense of strain and distress as a result of her fear of suffering and impending danger. Her hypochondria and self-acknowledged vulnerability renders her unable to enjoy an apparently peaceful and quiet old age, since she lives in a permanent state of alertness, trusting no intruders, and rejecting any interaction with those outside her shabby home.

The tiny derelict apartment in which she barricades herself behind a permanently locked door is presented as an extension of her fragile body, insofar as an initial tracking shot displays her neglected abode, with unkempt floors, dilapidated furniture, and half-boarded windows which expose Wanda to cold and snow as if she were virtually living in the open air. Wanda's frail body remains at the mercy of external perils that may finally put an end to her life in the same way as her derelict apartment is exposed to the inclemency of the bad weather. A contractor hired to demolish her home feels stunned upon discovering that someone is still living under such conditions and even deems her half-mad, as the place has been condemned and all the surrounding buildings have already been destroyed. Facing Wanda's reluctance to abandon her dwelling in spite of its imminent destruction, the contractor seems to establish further connections between Wanda's tampered abode and her fragile body, as he states that "when a building is old, it's dangerous. It's gotta come down to make room for a new one. That's life, lady. Old make room for the new

[...] A big tree falls and new ones grow right out of the same ground. Old animals die and young ones take their places. Even people step aside when it's time." Nevertheless, paying no heed to the contractor's warnings, Wanda intends to stay in her condemned basement room even if it is bound to be demolished, just as she holds on to her flimsy existence although she perceives that her final curtain will also come down soon.

In contrast, Wanda is gradually depicted as an inherently warmhearted and caring aging woman who renounces her sense of prudence if it is for the sake of helping others. As a close-up of her horrified face denotes, Wanda awakes in utter terror upon hearing some gunshots and the gasping voice of a young man asking her to come to his aid and disturb her isolation. Given her apprehensive nature, she double-checks that her door is properly locked before she dares to lay eyes upon Harold Beldon, a helpless attractive young officer in black, played by Robert Redford, who is lying wounded outside her apartment. His imploring cries for help pose an ethical issue when he declares that, unless she helps him, he will surely die. His relentless appeals not only force Wanda to conquer her fears, but also to face an existentialist dilemma, as she is well aware that the act of helping the man to save his life may be at the risk of exposing herself to death. In spite of her initial aversion, Wanda finally agrees to open the door of her apartment and nurse the wounded officer. Amazed that she is still alive after establishing contact with the stranger, Wanda discloses the reason for leading such a secluded existence and living in constant fear. To the young man's puzzlement, who finds the aging woman unreasonable and rather eccentric, Wanda admits that she feels in constant awe of meeting Mr. Death again and recounts the first time that she encountered him, which marked the advent of her old age:

> I was on a bus. There was an old woman sitting in front of me, knitting. Socks, I think. There was something about her face. I felt I knew her. Then this young man got on. There were empty seats, but he sat down beside her. He didn't say anything but... his being there upset her. He seemed like a nice young man. When she dropped her yarn, he picked it up. Right in front of me. He held it up to her. I saw their

fingers touch. He got out at the next stop. When the bus reached the end of the line... she was dead.

Ever since this epiphanic event, Wanda has protected herself from the lingering presence of Death, which is personified surprisingly by a young man who keeps on shifting his appearance and nobody, except herself, can see. Wanda explicitly acknowledges that aged people are able to spot Mr. Death, whereas young individuals may still perceive his presence, but not so clearly. She thus recognizes him owing to the fact that, to use her own words, she is "getting older" and feels her time is "coming." Upon recounting this event, ironically, Wanda subtly acknowledges her close attachment to "the old woman" on the bus, but she fails to establish a corresponding connection between the "nice young man" whom she identified as an embodiment of Death and the wounded officer that she has recently allowed into her house.

Nostalgically, looking back to her youth, Wanda recollects that she used to love being outdoors and basking in the sunlight, as opposed to her current self-imposed enclosure in old age, which urges her to lead a nearly vampiric existence, subsisting in the dark and detaching herself from the reality outside her apartment. Her metaphorical characterization as a vampire is also made effective by means of a close-up shot of her faltering hand reaching out to the timid, but warm, rays of sun shining across her half-boarded window, as if she were afraid of the light. Nonetheless, Wanda is not the only one who shares some of the archetypal features of the vampire, among which Anna Chromik highlights nocturnal life-style, polymorphism, a black attire, and a lack of shadow (2016: 709), which also characterize Wanda's male guest. The officer has been sharing Wanda's isolation and turn for living in the dark owing to his fragile condition during convalescence. It is a result of Wanda's consent, as she finally agrees to let him in her apartment, that he enters her abode, as vampires usually do to seduce their victims. Moreover, when the contractor assumes that Wanda is an eccentric old lady suffering from some sort of mental disorder because she appears to be talking to herself, she finally grasps that no one else can see the male officer except herself, which leads her to gain insight into the young man's preternatural condition. To confirm Wanda's suspicions, Beldon urges her to look at his non-existing reflection in the mirror, which matches the vampire's distinguishing lack of shadow. Moreover, he also manages to shift his appearance in resemblance with the polymorphic nature of the vampire. Beldon's characterization not only adds to his resemblance with the Gothic archetype of the vampire, but also reveals that he is the presence that Wanda has been trying to avoid, since, despite his innocent-looking appearance, like the nice young man on the bus, Beldon truly stands for the personification of Death.

Given the fact that only Wanda is aware of Beldon's presence, that the mirror does not reflect back his image, and that they swap places as bedridden convalescents, Wanda and Beldon turn them into doubles of one another. Bearing in mind that Otto Rank describes the double as either "the messenger of death" or "a wish-defense against a dreaded eternal destruction" (1971: 86), this ambivalent role paves the way for interpreting the character of Beldon as either the preternatural incarnation of Death which is coming for Wanda's life in her old age or, rather, as the symbolic materialization of Wanda's fears of death which her unstable mind projects and reifies in order to cope with them. In spite of her initial reluctance, Wanda finally agrees to take Beldon's hand and a close-up of their clasped hands calls to mind Wanda's memories about "the old woman" and "the nice young man" approaching each other on the bus. Moreover, when Beldon addresses Wanda as "mother" while they are holding hands, the contractor's words about the old making room for the new are evoked once again, as the process comes full circle and past and present appear to blend in.

Despite Wanda's expected fears of suffering upon the advent of death, Beldon appeases her confirming that "what you feared would come like an explosion is like a whisper – what you thought was the end is the beginning," as he asks her to look at herself lying dead in her bed, where the male officer had been lying up to then, once she has abandoned the world of the living. Beldon and Wanda exit her apartment and move outside, as Wanda realizes that, as opposed to the gloomy picture of Death that she had entertained for long, Death truly grants her the freedom that she was deprived of in her life as a result of constant fear. According to Plantinga, "Nothing in the Dark" offers a surprise ending of elevation which contributes to improving the understanding of humanity through positive prospects (2009: 47). Ironically, it is thus hinted that, during the last stages of her life, Wanda endures a vampiric existence which only ceases when the fearful act of dying takes place.

As Zicree claims, "Nothing in the Dark" provides "a thoughtful and moving statement on old age and the fear of death" (1992: 223), which subverts many conventional views about the end of life and approaches it as a natural process that should be embraced rather than rejected. When Wanda finally agrees to welcome the young man in her apartment, whereby she symbolically accepts to give in to Mr. Death, her life takes a turn for the better, and all her anxieties vanish once she envisions death as a sort of liberation from her cloistered existence.

Conventional depictions which characterize Death as a source of dread and terror are left behind in favor of portraying the end of life in an eminently positive light. In contrast with customary characterizations of Death as a gloomy and emaciated woman, as a temptress or female vampire, Beldon is rather depicted as a young man, whom James Taylor even describes as "pleasant, mild-mannered, and handsome" (2009: 172), hence contributing to forging the image of Death as an apparently innocent and approachable figure and, as Timothy Shary and Nancy McVittie claim (2016, 187), anticipating contemporary filmic depictions of Death embodied by attractive, albeit deceitful, young men. As Rod Serling's voice-over finally concludes at the end of the episode, Wanda discovers that "there was nothing in the dark that wasn't there when the lights were on," hence subverting the customary interpretation of Death as a horrifying figure that comes to haunt mortals and condemn them to an afterlife existence in complete darkness.

Away with Grandma: In Awe of the Beloved Departed in "Long Distance Call"

"Long Distance Call" also tackles death in old age, albeit it is portrayed in a more disturbing way in comparison with the optimistic prospects offered in "Nothing in the Dark." Its script was written by William Idelson and Charles Beaumont, the latter being considered second only to Serling in the number of *Twilight Zone* scripts produced and his narratives were characterized by "a strong morbidity and almost clinical fascination with the horrific" (Zicree 1992: 74). This episode portrays the last days of Grandma Bayles, played by Lili Darvas, who lives with her son, Chris, her daughter-in-law, Sylvia, and her grandson, Billy, to whom Grandma feels particularly attached, as is shown when Billy turns five and the family gather together to celebrate the birthday of the youngest member in the family. Although Grandma Bayles is at first depicted as noticeably frail and weak, she also represses some whimsical and even possessive traits which betray a strong personality, even though these turns are mostly attributed to the effects of illness or medication. "Long Distance Call" calls into question the widespread cultural image of the granny as an inherently benevolent and tender-hearted relative, insofar as, following her death, her spirit appears to be willing to hold on to life and exert a malignant influence on the most beloved, but also most vulnerable, member of the family, her grandson Billy. Grandma's ghostly presence extends after death, when she talks to her grandson by means of the toy phone she gave him as a present for his birthday, thus evincing her reluctance to sever the intimate bond that ties them together. Nevertheless, as James Taylor argues, the lengthy conversations that take place between Grandma and Billy on his toy phone, even after she has departed, may also address the child's process of coping with grief and coming to terms with death at such a young age and, to that end, he appears to concoct the strategy of talking to her late granny from 'the other side' (2009: 175). Grandma's lingering spirit may thus respond to Billy's own willingness not to let go off her out of love, owing to his inability to understand the actual meaning of death as a child.

Grandma's present, a toy phone, turns into a magic token, which leads Stanyard to categorize this episode as among those which resort to enchanted objects (2007: 53) whereby 'the marvelous' is granted entry and contributes to subverting the audience's expectations and distorting culturally assumed notions about life and death. In this case, the toy phone gradually turns into a case of demonic possession through which Grandma exerts her malignant influence on Billy so that he can join her in death and hold complete dominion over his young grandson. This episode thus addresses illness and death in old age, the stifling dominion that the old may hold over the young, and the reluctance of elders to give in to death. In particular, the character of Grandma Bayles fits within the subgenre that Miller and Bowdoin van Riper denominate as 'hag horror,' in which deranged older women are capable of exerting psychological and physical abuse on those around them (2019: 4). In addition, though, since this narrative also caters for an ambivalent interpretation, it also addresses the process of mourning and coming to terms with grief upon facing the death of aged relatives.

As Chivers contends, the aging body is generally associated with illness and disability, insofar as "old age is believed to indicate (at the very least) ill health, and ill health often visually appears in the form of the disabled body" (2011: 8). In the initial sequence of this episode, Grandma Bayles needs help to go down the stairs in order to join the family on Billy's birthday, thus evincing that she can hardly walk, she is dependent, and she is often short of breath, which is further emphasized when her son reminds her doctor's orders not to exert herself and that, as soon as possible, she should go back to her room to have some rest. Grandma Bayles is initially characterized as a loving, wrinkled, and soft-spoken granny, with her gray-hair tied in a low bun and wearing a black cardigan topped with an antique cameo which bespeaks of former times. Nonetheless, her fragile appearance contrasts with some outbursts of character that unveil a strong-minded and even cranky personality. When her son Chris reminds her that she should return to her room soon, she retorts that, "I always follow the rules of the house except when I don't agree with them" and, when she is prevented from cutting the cake not to exhaust herself, she objects, proclaiming that "you think I'm too old to cut the cake – when I'm that old you take the shovel and dig the hole." Despite her declining health, Grandma Bayles thus displays a strong will, as she would not miss her grandson's birthday for the world owing to the special relationship that unites them and from which Billy's parents often feel excluded.

The solid complicity between Grandma and grandson turns them into playmates and evokes the cultural trope of old age construed as second childhood, which envisions the aged as childlike and reverting back into children, thus exposing their dependency, but also blurring the age gap conventionally established between these two life stages, which emphasizes the cyclical, instead of linear, quality of aging. According to Jenny Hockey and Allison James, the traditional link of old age with childhood involves that the hegemony of adulthood remains unchallenged (1995: 138), as children and the aged are often subjugated in contrast with parents in the social stratum. Nonetheless, in "Long Distance Call," this cultural assumption is reversed, as the close-knit bond that ties Grandma Bayles and Billy together condemns his parents to ostracism.

Grandma's portrayal comprises traits pertaining to different Gothic archetypes which accentuate her ambivalence as a character initially depicted as a weak and warm-hearted granny. Before Billy blows out the candles on his birthday cake, at Grandma's request, he makes a wish and discloses it only to her, as she argues, in front of his parents, that "that's a secret between him and me." Grandma also urges Billy to open her present first when his parents are about to offer theirs and, upon displaying a toy telephone as her gift, she remarks it is "a telephone for us so that you can always talk to your grandma even when she is not here." Grandma's words about wishes and gifts conjure up the image of an aging fairy for Billy, even though her blunt possessive ways with her grandson in front of his parents also call to mind the fairy-tale character of the witch. In spite of her frail condition, before returning upstairs to the quietness of her room, Grandma gathers enough strength to express her fondness for her grandson, stating that "he gave me life again – to an old woman good for nothing, no more but to complain, he held out his hands to me and... made me alive." The metaphorical process of rejuvenation to which she refers is reminiscent of that of a vampire, who nourishes on the youth to prolong its existence in spite of its intrinsically old age.

The toy phone that Grandma gives Billy for his birthday acquires symbolic connotations as the link that ties both caller and recipient reinforces the close relationship established between Grandma and grandson, which she intends to extend even after her death. The toy phone turns into a devilish gift whereby Grandma will continue exerting control over Billy, as he begins to act as if he were possessed by a demonic spirit that urges him to hurt himself. Grandma's possessive and jealous nature is revealed on her deathbed, as she is no longer able to recognize her own son, Chris, stating that "my son was taken away by a woman," that is, Sylvia, Billy's mother, and pointing out that "this is my son, now, Billy." Even if Chris dismisses his mother's eerie words as a result of the effects of the medicine she is taking to soothe the pain, before dying, Grandma pleads to Billy, "I will be so lonely – I wish you could go with your Grandma," adding "far away, Billy – together, the two of us, just you and me." Her words carry some creepy connotations, since being together necessarily implies Billy's premature death. Grandma's wish on her deathbed calls to mind Billy's wish on his birthday, which symbolically marks her transition from her benevolent role as a fairy to her wicked part as a witch.

Billy seems to live in a trance once Grandma has passed away. Sylvia suspects that her son's almost catatonic state is due to the fact that Billy and Grandma were "too close," which may even hint subtly at a nearly incestuous relationship. Sylvia's words betray her jealousy, since, from Billy's perspective as a child, Grandma's omnipresence always relegated his own mother to the secondary role of the wicked stepmother in a fairy tale. In a deeply enigmatic scene, Billy beholds his reflection on the pond outside their house, which suggests some symbolic depersonalization, as Grandma gradually takes possession of the child. Billy's introspective nature suggests a precocious personality given his young age, particularly when his father asks him whether he can understand what death is and Billy nods confidently. As a precocious child, Billy looks young, but is aged inwardly, just as his grandmother looked aged, but exhibited a young spirit and strong will even in the last days of her life. Grandma and Billy symbolically lead a symbiotic existence, as her spirit imposes itself on Billy's soul and inhabits his body to make up for her physical absence. In the same way that Grandma's stubborn and childlike ways were disquieting, Billy's forlorn and precocious behavior as a child also proves deeply disturbing.

As Zicree argues, one of the most frightening implications of this episode lies in "the horrifying concept of a dead relative guiding a child toward suicide" (1992:193). Billy spends his days and nights talking on the toy phone and, upon his mother's insistence to tell her who he is talking to, Billy resolutely admits that he has been speaking to Grandma and that she feels so lonely that he wants him to come and play with her. In response to Grandma's demands, Billy begins to fall prey to a series of self-imposed misfortunes, which appear to be the result of Billy's being possessed by Grandma's spirit. However, since it is Billy who seems to be responsible for exposing himself to danger out of his will, his actions may also betray the ludicrous strategies of a child to cope with grief and his incapacity to accept his grandmother's death.

Although this narrative hints at a feasible interpretation, the sequence of events points to a fantastic, rather than rational, explanation. Even if Billy's mother is convinced that her son's strange behavior responds to his childish fantasies, when she wakes up in the middle of the night and overhears Billy talking on the toy phone, she picks up the receiver and realizes, to her horror, that Grandma's breathing can be heard on the other side. In spite of her initial benevolent appearance, which complies with the culturally constructed and popular image of the granny, Grandma's evil spirit is portrayed as willing to drag Billy with her after her death even if this may imply taking his life. When Billy jumps into the pond and medical resuscitation procedures prove of no avail, out of despair, his father talks to Grandma on the toy phone, stating: "Mother, you said Billy gave you life again – now you can give him life – if you really love him, let him live – give him back." Since it is Chris's symbolic exorcism rather than any medical treatment that saves Billy's life, it is eventually confirmed that Grandma's evil spirit had taken possession of the young child and had been responsible for the misfortunes that nearly cause his death.

Against all odds, this episode problematizes the image of the benevolent granny, as she is transformed into a demonic spirit even capable of hurting her own kin owing to her unquenchable possessive and selfish character. The portrayal of Grandma Bayles complies with the characters of evil older women that Miller and Bowdoir van Riper refer to as being initially presented as sympathetic victims whose strange behavior may be due to the fact that they can no longer exert control over their minds and bodies, although it is later revealed that something more sinister may be responsible for their eccentric conduct (2019: 7). As a character, Grandma Bayles calls to mind 'the monstrous feminine,' to use Barbara Creed's term, which endorses the connection between monstrosity and aging women, and is indicative of patriarchal anxieties about the female body in old age, thus conjuring ancestral fears of predatory females whose released instincts are considered particularly repulsive in their later years.

Conclusion

These four narratives display classic elements pertaining to the Gothic genre, in terms of settings, archetypal characters, and atmosphere which pave the way for the sinister to make its appearance. Isolated houses, ancient manors, wild landscapes, shabby basements, and cemeteries are locations in which the plot unfolds. Characters in these episodes such as Elva's fiancé, Anne Henderson, the young officer, Wanda Dunn, and Grandma Bayles are portrayed through features which are suggestive of Gothic archetypes. These characters are evocative of the zombie whose abject body becomes alive, the ghost who returns to avenge itself, the double who arises as a wise advisor and a reminder of death, the witch who threatens to repeal the spell of an apparently mesmerizing life, the vampire who wants to defy death but leads a life-in-death existence, and the demonic presence that alienates the familiar and must be exorcised. The creepy atmosphere in these narratives also contributes to creating a lingering sense of tension and strain by means of resorting to cold weather, storms, dark abodes, claustrophobia, decay, and a lingering feeling of helplessness and uncertainty.

In addition to displaying evident Gothic elements, these episodes are also thematically united insofar as they all explore fears and anxieties arising from the process of aging and the advent of old age. "Night Call" addresses fears related to aging badly, such as illness, dependence on others, loneliness and, particularly, guilty memories from the past. In "Spur of the Moment," the dual structure on which the narrative is constructed tackles the prejudices against old age, while it also suggests feelings of regret in later years as a result of a careless and irresponsible youth. "Nothing in the Dark" addresses the dread of death which leads Wanda to develop a selfish and even antisocial character as a result of extreme fear and apprehension during the last stages of life. In "Long Distance Call," the death of the oldest member in the family paves the way to explore grief at the death of our beloved ones, but also to suggest the uncanny influence that obstinate and possessive elders may still exert on those relatives who outlive them.

Given the ambivalent nature that characterizes the horror genre and the idiosyncratic 'twilight' resolutions which became a trademark of the series, these four narratives evoke culturally assumed images of aging and old age which are gradually subverted and ultimately called into question. By means of a carefully-crafted narratological structure that plays with the audience's expectations and resorts to socially-established dictates about aging and widespread representations of the aged in popular fiction, conventional portrayals of elders are first evoked, subsequently problematized, and eventually disrupted. Drawing on Carroll's terminology about tales of dread, which comprise narratives that rely on poetic justice (2009, 29), "Night Call" and "Spur of the Moment" would fit this category, inasmuch as, in their later years, Elva Keene and Anne Henderson are respectively punished for the sins of their youth. Although Elva is first portrayed as a victim, her wicked deeds are eventually revealed, whereas, Anne's aging self is initially depicted as a source of the abject, but whose intentions ultimately prove to be good. To use Plantinga's terms, some episodes offer a change of prospects, as is the case with "Night Call," in which the mysterious caller turns out to be Elva's late fiancé who unveils her wicked deeds in spite of her frail appearance in old age, while, in "Long Distance Call," loving Grandma Bayles reveals her possessive personality as her evil spirit comes back to life. Conversely, other narratives rather propose a change of frame whereby the assumed picture of reality is reversed. In "Spur of the Moment, the aging woman who terrifies Anne happens to be her aged double who chases her in order to prevent her from making a mistake in youth whose penalties she will have to pay in her old age. Similarly, in "Nothing in the Dark," Wanda Dunn's deeply-ingrained assumptions of death as terrifying are reversed, insofar as death is unusually portrayed as the visit of a handsome young man.

In some episodes, owing to dramatic irony, the spectator is more knowledgeable than the characters themselves, whereas, in other cases, important information about the character is upheld from the audience with the purpose of rendering this change of prospects effective. In "Night Call", viewers remain in a disadvantaged position in relation to Elva, its aged protagonist, since they remain ignorant of the wicked deed in her past. By contrast, in "Spur of the Moment", through a display of dramatic irony, young Anne is oblivious of the identity of the terrifying older woman who haunts her, whereas the audience is aware that the older woman in Anne herself. Some narratives rely on deflating surprises, which accentuate a rather pessimistic perspective, as happens in "Long Distance Call," whereby Grandma Bayles transforms from an apparently caring grandmother into an evil spirit, whereas other narratives resort to elevating surprises which make the episode end in a positive note, as happens in "Nothing in the Dark" and its rather alluring, and innovative, portrayal of death. Finally, some of these horror narratives emphasize their inherent ambiguity by means of offering open endings that foster different interpretations. In "Night Call," the calls that disturb Elva's lonely days in old age can be interpreted as either the punishment her fiancé wishes to inflict on her or the result of her guilty memories, while, in "Long Distance Call," Grandma Bayle's return as an evil spirit may be owing to her wicked nature, which she had been repressing for life or, rather, as a result of her grandson's emotional response upon coming to terms with the death of his beloved grandmother.

The narratological elements displayed in these narratives promote critical thinking, to use Plantinga's term (2009: 48), thus calling into question established sets of beliefs, ideological frameworks, and cultural assumptions in relation to old age. As the plot unfolds, conventional representations of elders are gradually transformed in favor of exposing an ambivalent portrayal of old age which unveils the intricacies of the discourses of aging and openly explore latent, and even repressed, fears and anxieties about this later stage of life. Horror, thus, arises as an appropriate genre to explore social phobias about aging and old age in order to destabilize them and subvert them, ultimately revealing that stereotypical and social perceptions of old age are culturally constructed. As Carroll argues, the paradox of horror is that spectators are willing to experience fear as the price to indulge in the pleasures of narratives that nourish the belief of revealing the unknown (1990: 159). The horror narratives about aging from *The Twilight Zone* are rooted in this promise of disclosing interstices of eternal truths in relation to human and philosophical aspects of life and death. After all, as Clayton Johnson, writer of "Nothing in Dark" contends, *The Twilight Zone* "compares with any great work, from the Holy Bible almost, to the *Iliad* and the *Odyssey*" (Stanyard 2007: 177), given the transcendent issues it explores in all its episodes which all together make up an epic work that represents a milestone in American popular fiction and still exerts enormous influence on contemporary films of fantasy and horror.

Author Bio

Marta Miquel-Baldellou holds an International PhD in comparative literature. She is a postdoctoral researcher and a member of the Centre of literatures and cultures in English at the University of Lleida (Catalonia, Spain). Her field of research revolves around Gothic fiction, aging studies, and film theory. She also works as a translator and a writer.

Works Cited

Basting, Anne Davis (1998): The Stages of Age: Performing Age in Contemporary American Culture, Michigan: University of Michigan Press.

Beaumont, Charles and William Idelson (1961): "Long Distance Call." In: James Sheldon (dir.), Rod Serling's The Twilight Zone, Second Season, CBS.

Boddy, William (1984): "Entering The Twilight Zone." In: Screen 25, pp. 98–108.

Carroll, Noël (1990): The Philosophy of Horror, London: Routledge.

Carroll, Noël (2009): "Tales of Dread in The Twilight Zone: A Contribution to Narratology." In: Noël Carroll and Lester H. Hunt (eds.), Philosophy in The Twilight Zone, Chichester: Wiley-Blackwell, pp. 26–38.

Chivers, Sally (2013): The Silvering Screen, Toronto: University of Toronto Press.

Covey, Herbert C. (1991): Images of Older People in Western Art and Society, New York: Praeger.

Creed, Barbara (1993): The Monstrous Feminine: Film, Feminism, and Psychoanalysis, New York: Routledge.

Gullette, Margaret Morganroth (2004): Aged by Culture, Chicago: University of Chicago Press.

Hockey, Jenny and Allison James (1995): "Back to Our Futures: Imaging Second Childhood." In: Mike Featherstone and Andrew Wernick (eds.), Images of Aging: Cultural Representations of Later Life, London and New York: Routledge, pp. 135–148.

Johnson, George Clayton (1962): "Nothing in the Dark." In: Lamont Johnson (dir.), Rod Serling's The Twilight Zone, Third Season, CBS.

Chromik, Anna (2016): "Vampire Fiction." In: William Hughes, David Punter, and Andrew Smith (eds.), The Encyclopedia of the Gothic, Chichester: Wiley-Blackwell, pp. 707–711.

King, Stephen (2000): Danse Macabre, London: Warner Books.

Kristeva, Julia (1982): Powers of Horror: An Essay on Abjection, Leon S. Roudiez (trans.), New York: Columbia University Press.

Matheson, Richard (1964): "Night Call" (based on Matheson's short story "Long Distance Call"). In: Jacques Tourneur (dir.), Rod Serling's The Twilight Zone, Fifth Season, CBS.

Matheson, Richard (1964): "Spur of the Moment." In: Elliot Silverstein (dir.), Rod Serling's The Twilight Zone, Fifth Season, CBS.

Matheson, Richard (2008): "Long Distance Call." In: Victor LaValle (ed.), The Best of Richard Matheson, New York: Penguin Classics, pp. 253–265. (Originally published as "Sorry, Right Number" in Beyond Fantasy Fiction in 1953).

Miller, Cynthia J. and A. Bowdoin van Riper (2019): "Introduction." In Cynthia J. Miller and A. Bowdoin van Riper (eds.), Elder Horror: Essays on Film's Frightening Images of Aging, Jefferson: McFarland, pp. 1–9.

Miquel-Baldellou, Marta (2016): "In the Twilight of Their Lives? Magical Objects as Serial Devices and Catalysts of Aging in The Twilight Zone." In: Maricel Oró-Piqueras and Anita Wohlmann (eds.), Serializing Age: Aging and Old Age in TV Series, Bielefeld: transcript, pp. 109–135.

Nolan, William F. (2009): "The Matheson Years: A Profile in Friendship." In: Stanley Wiater, Matthew R. Bradley and Paul Stuve (eds.), The Twilight and Other Zones: The Dark Worlds of Richard Matheson, New York: Citadel Press Books.

Plantinga, Carl (2009): "Frame Shifters: Surprise Endings and Spectator Imagination in The Twilight Zone." In: Noël Carroll and Lester H. Hunt (eds.), Philosophy in The Twilight Zone, Chichester: Wiley-Blackwell, pp. 39–57.

Rank, Otto (1971): Double: A Psychoanalytic Study, Harry Tucker, Jr. (ed.), Chapel Hill: The University of North Carolina Press.

Shary, Timothy and Nancy McVittie (2016): Fade to Gray: Aging in American Cinema, Austin: University of Texas Press.

Stanyard, Stewart T. (2007): Dimensions behind The Twilight Zone, Toronto: ECW Press.

Stevens, David (2010): The Gothic Tradition, Cambridge: Cambridge University Press.

Taylor, James S. (2009): "Nothing in the Dark: Deprivation, Death, and the Good Life." In: Noël Carroll and Lester H. Hunt (eds.), Philosophy in The Twilight Zone, Chichester: Wiley-Blackwell, pp. 171–186.

Todorov, Tzvetan (1975): The Fantastic: A Structural Approach to a Literary Genre, Richard Howard (trans.), Ithaca: Cornell University Press.

Walker, Barbara G. (1985): The Crone: Women of Age, Wisdom, and Power, New York: Harper and Row.
Woodward, Kathleen (1983): "Instant Repulsion: Decrepitude, the Mirror Stage, and the Literary Imagination." In: The Kenyon Review 5/4, pp. 43–66.
Woodward, Kathleen (2006): "Performing Age, Performing Gender." In: NWSA Journal 18/1, pp. 162–189.
Zicree, Marc Scott (1992): The Twilight Zone Companion, Los Angeles: Silman-James Press.

Uncanny Female Aging in Dahl's Horror

Ieva Stončikaitė[1]

Introduction

Getting older is one of the biggest contemporary fears or 'gerontophobia' and it is often associated with unease and anxieties (Woodward 1999; DeFalco 2010). Although there is increasing visibility of older adults on a global scale, old age continues to be stereotyped and gendered in contemporary western culture. During the last decades, there has been noticeable growth and attention given to the dynamics of aging from interdisciplinary approaches that go beyond the traditional field of gerontology. Age scholars have argued that gerontology needed cultural and humanities-related perspectives in order to enrich and expand gerontological knowledge and scientific approaches to later life, which cannot be measured or understood by empirical research alone (Hepworth 2000; Gullette 2004; Casado Gual et al. 2016; Oró-Piqueras/Falcus 2018; Barry/ Vibe Skagen 2020).

Literature, culture, and the arts not only mirror the established notions of old age, but can also reshape preconditioned beliefs about aging and even create different narratives about later life (Oró-Piqueras 2016). Hepworth highlights that "gerontologists occasionally draw on fiction to illustrate the findings of empirical research or to interweave gerontology and fiction in order to enhance our understanding of aging" (2000: 3). Relatedly, literature and character identification permit the readers to sympathize with specific characters and even experience some degree

[1] Pompeu Fabra University.

of 'narrative empathy' that may act as a stimulus to emotional responsiveness and as a consciousness-raising mechanism (Keen 2007). And yet, there is not one specific research method or heuristic technique in literary studies of aging, as there is not one single experience of aging (Zeilig 2011). A literary approach does not give us clear answers to questions about old age, but rather helps reveal what aging implies socioculturally, politically, and individually from a life course perspective (Zeilig 2011; Kriebernegg 2015; Falcus 2016; Oró-Piqueras 2016).

This chapter contributes to interdisciplinary approaches to aging and shows how humanities-based perspectives can illuminate research into aging, ageism, and the socioculturally constructed images of later life. By merging literary age studies and the horror genre, it focuses on well-known British writer Roald Dahl's short story 'The Landlady,' first published in *The New Yorker* and later reprinted in the anthology *Kiss Kiss* (1960). By giving a special attention to the female protagonist, the chapter explores how different symbolic and gothic textual elements contribute to the narrative of decline and the negative notion of aging. In the story, later life is portrayed as a source of horror and evokes a fear of aging. Although Dahl's tale provides some hints that aging can be empowering and liberating for older women, the eerie and witchlike portrayal of the landlady proves that older age is enshrined in negative and even grotesque perceptions of later years. Dahl's narrative also reminds us that gender plays a crucial role in creating dominant master narratives of aging and cultural images of later life in popular cultural expressions (DeFalco 2010; de Medeiros 2016). The use of horror helps further expose the individual and societal fears of growing older and the challenges of female aging. Shedding light on Dahl's dark narrative from the perspective of age studies offers new vantage points from which to review the author's literary legacy and rethink the representations of female aging in popular literature.

Roald Dahl, the Master of Horror

Roald Dahl is, without a doubt, one of the most internationally successful and acclaimed masters of short stories for children and adults. His adult short story collections *Someone Like You* (1953), *Kiss, Kiss* (1960), and *Switch Bitch* (1974) were best-sellers in a market that was dominated by novels and autobiographies. Dahl's work was translated into many languages worldwide, making him a celebrity figure (Warren 1988; Mehmi 2014). The writer's famous short story 'The Landlady' also resembles Ernest Bloch's novel *Psycho* (1959), which was adapted into Alfred Hitchcock's pivotal 1960 film of the same name (Mehmi 2014). Even though Dahl is never included in the list of Gothic writers, except for his children stories, which are commonly defined as gothic, his adult tales cannot be easily categorized, and are often described as macabre, supernatural, uncanny, bizarre, mad, and threatening the social order (West 1990, 1992; Sohier 2011; Mehmi 2014; Van Haegenborgh 2015). His adult short stories contain explicit savage and fantasy elements, perverse and unpredictable deaths, intense insanity of his characters, and ironic unexpected endings. Dahl's most popular short stories fuse different stylistic, thematic, and formal elements that reflect "a vivid eye for detail, an elegance of writing and a real virtuosity in plotting" that are derived from the American short story tradition initiated by Edgar Allan Poe, O. Henry, and Ernest Hemingway (Mehmi 2014: 2–3; Van Haegenborgh 2015).

Ghastly, violent, grotesque, and mysterious features in Dahl's suspense fiction are used to project the deepest fears and taboos that society tends to mask or ignore. At the same time, gothic elements and settings make the readers question reality in ways that realistic or mimetic fiction could not do (Fabrizi 2016, 2018). While fantasy tends to provide escape from the mundane existence, horror offers a more profound analysis of the unfamiliar and can even lead to catharsis (Fabrizi 2018). The creation of an anxiety-and-suspense filled atmosphere, fused with exaggeration and mystery, guides the readers towards a climatic effect that is aimed to evoke a feeling of unease, and to question conventional reality and the dark side of humanity (Van Haegenborgh 2015: 65). Relatedly, horror texts and subversive meanings allow for "a safe exploration of the feelings of fear and danger" and offer a possibility "to wallow in the forbidden – to take joy in destruction and the normally unacceptable or unthinkable" (Brock-Servais 2018: 18). Such narratives also represent not only individual but also societal concerns of repressed, marginalized, or disadvantaged individuals, and show the limits of humanity (Clemens 1999). Contrary to common belief, horror is not aimed at scaring the readers, but rather at moving them out of their comfort zones and exposing real-world issues and individual struggles (Brock-Servais 2018; Ostenton 2018). As Brock-Servais argues, supernatural and scary figures in horror literature often represent "mindless conformity, a fear of contagion or pandemic, anxiety concerning the underclass (the masses), the loss of identity, or a critique of consumerism" (2018: 23). Horror literature functions as a mirror that reflects our inner desires and fears by providing spaces to critically rethink our understanding of the world and human nature.

Although Dahl's fiction, especially his children's literature, has been under a great deal of scrutiny and received more acclaim than criticism (Warren 1988; West 1992; Mehmi 2014), his adult stories did not receive much attention. Moreover, his adult fiction has not been approached through the lens of age studies, which, as will be shown, leads to novel readings and interpretations of his writings and fills a certain research gap. In 'The Landlady', horror serves as a means to empower the older character and challenge the conventional notions of old age as a stage of frailty, asexuality, and dependence (Gullette 2004). Yet, the landlady's emancipation is enshrined in irrationality and grotesqueness, reinforcing the stereotypical image of older women as witches, crones, female monsters, or women gone wild (Greer 1991). Dahl's representation of female aging is controversial and further underpins the negative notions of later life that emphasize contemporary fears of old age and getting older.

The Witchlike Landlady

Roald Dahl begins his sinister short story by depicting a young man, Billy Weaver, who travels alone in search of work, and is extremely excited about the new opportunities that await him. As he walks through the unfamiliar city of Bath in miserable and "deadly cold" weather, he decides to lodge in a charming B&B hotel (Dahl 2004: e10). The boarding house seems like a cozy and inviting place, decorated with yellow chrysanthemums, – flowers often used in funerals in many parts of Europe. As the boy lingers outside, the door is suddenly opened by a "terribly nice" woman who offers him a cheap price for lodgings (Dahl 2004: e12). Although she is between 45 and 50 years old, which is not considered old in contemporary society, we only see her through the focalization of a young man to whom anyone over 40 might seem quite old. Billy Weaver is informed that there have only been two previous guests – Mr. Christopher Mulholland and Mr. Gregory W. Temple –, who, apparently, have never left the hotel. The boy realizes that he has seen their names in a newspaper mentioning their odd disappearance. Yet, he is not suspicious and is even amused by the lady's strange behavior. In fact, the boy decides that she is not harmful but rather "a kind and generous soul" (Dahl 2004: e14). The landlady serves her new guest a cup of tea and, by scrutinizing his body, compliments him on his youthful looks and his unblemished body. She also reveals that she is a skilled taxidermist and has stuffed her dead pets, a dachshund and a parrot, which Billy Weaver thought to be alive. At this very moment, the boy realizes that his tea tastes of bitter almonds and inquires of the landlady if there have been any other guests except for the two visitors, to which she smilingly replies: "No, my dear" [...]. Only you" (Dahl 2004: e18). Although Dahl leaves an open ending, the readers are given enough hints to understand that Billy Weaver's fate will be that of the stuffed pets and the previous guests.

By killing a young man, the landlady seems to rebel against the gendered narrative of decline (Gullette 2004) and double marginalization, which further exclude and ignore older women's voices and their participation in society. Through the merciless and monstrous act of murder she might have been looking not only for revenge, but also for more visibility, which had been denied to her as a nameless aging woman. Driven by a feeling of anger, loneliness, and impotence, the heroine uses violence as a means to make herself more powerful and visible, and threatens the status quo. The eerie ending to Dahl's work can be read as women's revenge on sexism, ageism, dominant master discourses, and societal expectations.

The use of horror elements in the story also allows for the archetypical witch figure to re-emerge freely and demonstrate her power and skills. In fact, it is common in horror literature to portray the figure of a witch, which, in popular culture and folklore, represents malevolent forces, the murder of children and young adults, and the use of poison and potions to kill or curse people (Hutton 2017). Crystallized during the Early Modern period in Europe, the image of the witch continues to embody the eeriness of the unknown, fearful, or unreasonable. Witches have a distinguished history in western memory, which grants them a special position in society that evokes respect mingled with fear (Greer 1991). Moreover, the witch very often functions as a scapegoat in society at a time when a sound explanation to strange phenomena or occurrences cannot be given, which makes her the 'other' or the outsider. The fact that witches do not adhere to any of the institutionalized religions also positions them in a category of rebels who reject prevailing moral codes and conventional standards, and go against established rules and regulations. However, the witch also continues to denote an ambiguous and conflicting character that not only subverts the status quo and challenges misogynist symbols, but also proves problematic for feminism and age studies. As Germaine Buckley argues, "[w]itches as monstrous older women harbouring an unnatural desire for power is one facet of a Western ideology that situates women as outsiders to power" that has been represented as illegitimate and excluding since classical antiquity (2019: 29). Thus, it is not clear whether the witch figure empowers (older) women or hints at patriarchal fears about female power and sexuality (Berenstein 1990; Germaine Buckley 2019).

Macabre Female Sexuality

The identification of the lady with the witch figure also points to sexual transgressions, primal desires, and a relationship with evil forces or the Devil, as documented in many treatises on witchcraft and witch-hunts, such as the *Malleus Maleficarum* (1486). Even if the sexual desire of the landlady is not explicit, the readers can find subtle hints that suggest that she indulges in necrophiliac practices once she has successfully performed the art of taxidermy (and witchcraft) upon her young innocent victims. The heroine states that she is always prepared to meet young charming men and greet them with pleasure:

> But I'm always ready. Everything is always ready day and night in this house just on the off-chance that an acceptable young gentleman will come along. And it is such a pleasure, my dear, such a very great pleasure when now and again I open the door and I see someone standing there who is just exactly right (Dahl 2004: e13).

Although it may be argued that the identification of the landlady with the witch may point to female freedom and emancipation from the desired reproductive function aimed at demographic growth and social development, the heroine does not deny her sexual urges. Although she is freed from the male gaze imbued with sexual desire (Greer 1991), she manifests her sexuality through the macabre and grotesque treatment of Billy Weaver's dead body, which may be read as suppressed desires of the 'other' who is alienated from the outside world. Her red fingernails also symbolize sexuality and, thus, challenge the idea of asexual older women, which is in line with the discourse of active or successful aging that stresses the importance of sex and sexuality in later life (Walz 2002; Berdychevsky/Nimrod 2017). The landlady's desire to disrupt the social order and defy male dominance might also stem from a misogynistic portrayal of post-menopausal women as no longer attractive and sexually appealing, which leads one to think they are frustrated. Although, in recent decades, new shifts in understanding female sexuality and sex have contributed to perceiving the menopause in a more positive light (Sandberg 2015), the eerie depiction of the landlady points to disrespectful identifications of post-menopausal women with old witches. In Dahl's narrative, the image of a sexual older woman does not contribute to counteracting gerontophobia, but further highlights ageism and stigma inherent in the grotesque embodiment of the 'crazy old lady' or a hag. In fact, the origin of the word 'hag' (Old English) signifies a witch, sorceress, enchantress or a repulsive older woman, which reinforces the idea of fear of the power of older women.

It is also worth mentioning that Dahl's fiction and his use of unprecedented sexual violence has frequently been described as misogynist, especially prominent in his short story collection *Switch Bitch* that features unadulterated pornographic fantasies and cruelty against women (Mehni 2004). Actually, the very title of this collection reveals sexist overtones, and four of the stories in *Switch Bitch* were originally published in *Playboy* between 1965 and 1974. However, even though sexist violence and macabre elements are common in many of Dahl's works, in 'The Landlady' these aspects are twisted. It is the aging woman who uses cruelty against innocent young men for her own pleasure and perverse sexual fantasies. Sohier (2011) points out that the inclusion of horror elements in the tale hinge on the Freudian idea of a death instinct in human behavior, and states that the death-drive and life-drive complement each other. In fact, the scholar argues that "the death instinct constitutes the drive *par excellence*" as it underlines "all the other drives that are subsumed under the word 'Eros'" (Sohier 2011: 2, emphasis in original). According to Freud, human sexuality is closely linked to the destructive power and eroticism that is expressed in sexual fantasies and dreams that may signal emotional disorders, neuroses, and inner conflicts. Dahl's tale shows that some secreted sexual desires might be frightening and manifest themselves in the strangest ways, such as taxidermy and the subtly implied necrophilic acts. The use of the macabre and horror in the story, hence, allows further exploration of different scenarios surrounding the complexities of human sexuality that, contrary to the popular belief, do not decline with age, but can acquire new forms of expression (Stončikaitė 2017). The eerie and slightly humorous culmination of the story is also a story of a desire for immortality, longevity, and rejuvenescence.

The Desire for Eternal Youth

In Dahl's work, an older woman is characterized as an evil and selfish witch that is obsessed with stopping the ravages of time. The resemblance of the landlady with the archetypical image of the witch not only points to her desire for eternal youth, but also signals the bodily decay, deformation, sagging, and vulnerability that comes with age.

As women grow older, they become more invisible and desexualized; however, aging becomes more visible on their bodies and, especially, their faces (Woodward 1991; Bordo 2003; Öberg 2003; Hurd-Clarke 2011; Furman 2013; Hurd-Clarke/Bennett 2015; Stončikaitė 2020). The fact that the female protagonist remains nameless in the story further reinforces the invisibility of older women and the idea of the eerie otherness of later life (Woodward 1991; DeFalco 2010).

In the story, the landlady scrutinizes youthful Billy Weaver's body and is excited about its perfection: "her blue eyes travelled slowly all the way down the length of Billy's body, to his feet, and then up again" (Dahl 2004: e13). She is constantly keeping an eye on the boy to ensure that she captures his flawless beauty in order to perform the sadistic act of taxidermy and, in so doing, to keep the young man's impeccability forever: "Billy knew that she was looking at him. Her body was half-turned towards him, and he could feel her eyes resting on his face, watching him over the rim of her teacup" (Dahl 2004: e16-17). Billy Weaver becomes the sexualized object of desire whose body is scrutinized and subject to transgressive violence leading to macabre death, after which his stuffed corpse will be used for visual delectation of the lady (Mehni 2004). In fact, all three victims are young men in the prime of their lives: "they were extraordinarily handsome, both of them, I can promise you that. They were tall and young and handsome, my dear, just exactly like you" (Dahl 2004: e15). The landlady thinks that seventeen is the most marvelous age for it is positioned on the threshold of becoming eighteen, which officially marks the stepping into adulthood and the loss of innocence:

> 'Seventeen!' she cried. 'Oh, it's the perfect age! Mr Mulholland was also seventeen. But I think he was a trifle shorter than you are, in fact I'm sure he was, and his teeth weren't quite so white. You have the most beautiful teeth, Mr Weaver, did you know that? (Dahl 2004: e17).

Although one of her three victims, Mr. Temple, was older, he still preserved youthful beauty, softness, and handsomeness:

> 'Mr Temple, of course, was a little older,' she said [...]. 'He was actually twenty-eight. And yet I never would have guessed it if he hadn't told me, never in my whole life. There wasn't a blemish on his body.' 'A what?' Billy said. 'His skin was just like a baby's' (Dahl 2004: e17).

Sohier suggests that "a desire for the perfection of the skin, the fascination of the body" is closely linked to "a desire for whiteness, the whiteness of teeth and, in the same breath, with an insistent apprehension of age and aging" (2011: 9). The fact that the landlady "performs taxidermy not only on her pets but also on unwary young men, makes her into an uncanny woman, a figure of death, a representation of the death-drive" (Sohier 2011: 2). Although, by stuffing Billy Weaver's body, the lady champions the eternal beauty and youthful innocence that cannot be found in older age, her sinister acts are not empowering as they manifest irrationality, insanity, and the decline that comes with age. Even if through the performance of taxidermy the aging heroine gains power over youth and preserves her male victims' youthfulness, her resemblance to the witch further reinforces the notion of aging women as evil and threatening the social order and patriarchal domain.

Conclusions

Roald Dahl's work has not been approached from the lens of age studies – one of the aims of this chapter was to fill this research gap. In the short story 'The Landlady,' female aging is presented as a source of horror and grotesqueness. And yet, the very use of horror in the light of literary age studies helps expose the often silenced and tabooed aspects of female aging and the overriding fears of older age. In his depiction of the female character, Dahl shows different clichés about aging women, such as witches, hags, crones, or women gone mad. The landlady is not an absolute outsider or scapegoat; however, her portrayal as an evil and rebellious aging woman does not grant her enough agency beyond rebellion, thus hindering the production of a counter-narrative to the master narrative of decline (Gullette 2014). Although she is given a voice to share her desires and vulnerability, ageism and sexism continue to be inherent in the grotesque embodiment of the crazy murderer in a lonely house. Her macabre acts display the problematic and controversial image of a witch or the 'other,' which is deeply rooted in many cultural representations of older women. The fact that the landlady goes unpunished for her unprecedented and anxiety-ridden cruelty and necrophiliac fantasies further justifies misogynist views toward women, especially older women.

The chapter has also aimed to convey that the horror genre, sometimes considered inferior in comparison to more realistic and mimetic texts (Drout 2006; Fabrizi 2018), can serve as a tool to further explore individual and societal complexities and desires. Gothic and macabre elements help evoke deeper emotions that can lead to more critical readings of popular narratives and reveal how they shape our visions of the world and our identities (Ostenton 2018). As Mehmi argues, "Dahl's short story has gained its success because it functions cathartically as a deadening of pride, revenge, incestuous desire and rebellion and also as a social reconfiguration of being" (2014: 34). The use of horror allows for a safer exploration of our fears and anxieties, brings to light unvoiced, marginalized, and repressed individuals, and helps critically approach conventional truths by revealing societal and individual struggles (Clemens 1999; Brock-Servais 2018; Ostenton 2018). A closer analysis of how horror elements interact with gender relationships and the representations of aging in popular writings would enrich not only gerontological scholarship, but also feminist, horror, fantasy, age, queer studies, and beyond.

Ultimately, the study has attempted to show that a critical examination of how the images of older adults are created within popular culture is important in order not to reproduce age-related stereotypes, which may further exclude, denigrate, and marginalize older people (Goldman 2017). Henneberg, for instance, proposes writing texts that are "in active opposition to received patterns of ageism" and include more realistic portrayals of older age and older women (2010: 132, 133). Literature, popular cultural expressions, and the arts are powerful tools and extensions of sociocultural developments and individual stories that need to be told, shared, and heard in order to enable different narratives of growing up and growing older alike. More positive representations of older people are important because the stories we tell create the social imagery of older age and influence the ways we understand the life course. Examining popular texts from the age-studies perspective can help dislodge many stereotypical notions of aging and create other stories in which older women are given more roles besides the witch or the crazy and uncanny old lady.

Author Bio

Ieva Stončikaitė holds a PhD in Cultural & Literary Gerontology and English Studies (University of Lleida, Spain). She is currently a Post-doctoral Researcher and English literature lecturer at the Department of Humanities at Pompeu Fabra University (Barcelona). Her areas of academic focus include literary and cultural representations of ageing, medical humanities, dementia care and ethics, illness narratives, age-friendly higher education, and travel writing. Ieva is a member of the research group CELCA (Center for Literatures and Cultures in English, University of Lleida), a Board Member of ENAS (European Network in Ageing Studies) and the 'RN01_Ageing in Europe' ESA Network (European Sociological Association). She is also part of the Young Leaders Academy / Cohort 3 (EUTOPIA Alliance). Ieva has presented her research at numerous conferences, seminars, and guest lectures. Her articles appear in journals such as *The Gerontologist, Journal of Aging Studies, Educational Gerontology*, and *Life Writing*, as well as in edited collections published by Routledge and Palgrave.

Author's Note

This chapter is a shortened and modified version of an article "Roald Dahl's Eerie Landlady: A Macabre Tale of Aging" published in *Journal of Aging Studies* 62. Copyright Elsevier 2022.

Works Cited

Barry, Elizabeth/Vibe Skagen, Margery (2020): "Introduction: The Difference That Time Makes." In Elizabeth Barry/Margery Vibe Skagen (eds.), Literature and Ageing, D.S. Brewer, pp. 1–15.

Berdychevsky, Liz/Nimrod, Galit (2017): "Sex As Leisure In Later Life: A Netnographic Approach." In: Leisure Sciences 39, pp. 224–243.

Berenstein, Rhona (1990): "Mommie Dearest: Aliens, Rosemary's Baby and Mothering." In: Journal of Popular Culture, 24/2, pp. 55–73.

Bordo, Susan (2003): Unbearable Weight: Feminism, Western Culture, and The Body, Berkeley, Los Angeles: University of California Press.

Brock-Servais, Rhona (2018): "Can We Redeem The Monster? Working With Contemporary Young Adult Horror Fiction In The College Classroom." In: Fabrizi, Mark A. (ed.), Horror Literature and Dark Fantasy. Critical Literacy Teaching Series: Challenging Authors and Genres, Leiden; Boston: Brill, pp. 17–29.

Casado Gual, Núria/Domínguez Rué, Emma/Worsfold, Brian (eds.) (2016): Literary Creativity and The Older Woman Writer: A Collection of Critical Essays, Bern: Peter Lang.

Clemens, Valdine (1999): The Return of The Repressed: Gothic Horror From Otranto To Alien, Albany, New York: SUNY Press.

Dahl, Roald (2004 [1960]): "The Landlady." *Kiss Kiss*. Penguin. E-book.

de Medeiros, Kate (2016): "Narrative Gerontology: Countering The Master Narratives of Aging." In: Narrative Works: Issues, Investigations, & Interventions 6/1, pp. 63–81.

Drout, Michael D. C. (2006): Lecture Series: Of Sorcerers and Men: Tolkien and The Roots of Modern Fantasy Literature, Prince Frederick (MD): Recorded Books, LLC.

Fabrizi, Mark A. (2016): "Introduction." In: Mark A. Fabrizi (ed.), Fantasy Literature: Challenging Genres, Rotterdam, the Netherlands: Sense Publishers.

Fabrizi, Mark A. (2018): "Introduction: Challenging Horror Literature and Dark Fantasy." In: Mark A. Fabrizi (ed.), Horror Literature and Dark Fantasy. Critical Literacy Teaching Series: Challenging Authors and Genres, Leiden; Boston: Brill, pp. 1–17.

Falcus, Sarah (2016): "Literature and Ageing." In Julia Twigg/Wendy Martin (eds.), Routledge Handbook of Cultural Gerontology, London and New York: Routledge, pp. 53–60.

Furman, Frida Kerner (2013): Facing The Mirror: Older Women and Beauty Shop Culture, New York: Routledge.

Germaine Buckley, Cloe (2019): "Witches, 'Bitches' or Feminist Trailblazers? The Witch In Folk Horror Cinema." In: Frances Kamm/Tamar Jeffers McDonald (eds.), Revenant: Creative and Critical Studies of The Supernatural. Gothic Feminisms, pp. 22–42.

Goldman, Marlene (2017): Forgotten: Narratives of Age-Related Dementia and Alzheimer's Disease In Canada, Montreal, Quebec: McGill-Queen's Press.

Greer, Germaine (1991): The Change: Women, Aging and The Menopause, London: Hamish Hamilton.

Gullette, Margaret Morganroth (2004): Aged By Culture, Chicago: University of Chicago Press.

Henneberg, Sylvia (2010): "Moms Do Badly, But Grandmas Do Worse: The Nexus of Sexism and Ageism In Children's Classics." In: Journal of Aging Studies 24, pp. 125–134.

Hepworth, Mike (2000): Stories of Aging, Buckingham: Open University.
Hurd-Clarke, Laura (2011): Facing Age Women Growing Older In Anti-Aging Culture, Lanham, Md: Rowman & Littlefield.
Hurd-Clarke, Laura/Bennett, Erica V. (2015): "Gender, Aging, and Appearance." In Julia Twigg/Wendy Martin (eds.), Routledge Handbook of Cultural Gerontology, London; New York: Routledge, pp. 133–141.
Hutton, Ronald (2017): The Witch: A History of Fear From Ancient Times To The Present, New Haven; London: Yale University Press.
Keen, Suzanne (2007): Empathy and The Novel, Oxford, New York: Oxford University Press.
Kriebernegg, Ulla (2015): "Literary Gerontology: Understanding Aging As A Lifelong Process Through Cultural Representation." In: The Gerontologist 55 (Issue Suppl. 2) 839.
Mehmi, Suneel S. (2014): "Understanding The Significance and Purpose of Violence In The Short Stories of Roald Dahl." In: PSYART: A Hyperlink Journal For The Psychological Study of The Arts 18, pp. 205–229.
Öberg, Peter (2003): "Images Versus Experience of The Aging Body." In: Christopher A. Faircloth (ed.), Aging Bodies: Images and Everyday Experience, California: Altamira Press, pp. 103–132.
Oró-Piqueras, Maricel (2016): "The Loneliness of The Aging In Two Contemporary Novels." In: The Gerontologist 56/2, pp. 193–200.
Oró-Piqueras, Maricel/Falcus, Sarah (2018): "Approaches To Old Age: Perspectives From The Twenty-First Century." In: European Journal of English Studies, 22/1, pp. 1–12.
Ostenson, Jon (2018): "What If The Dragon Can't Be Defeated? Examining The Coming-of-Age Narrative In Neil Gaiman's Coraline." In Mark A. Fabrizi (ed.), Horror Literature and Dark Fantasy. Critical Literacy Teaching Series: Challenging Authors and Genres, Leiden; Boston: Brill, pp. 41–55.
Sandberg, Linn (2015): "Sex, Sexuality, and Later Life." In Julia Twigg/Wendy Martin (eds.), Routledge Handbook of Cultural Gerontology, London; New York: Routledge, pp. 218–226.
Sohier, Jacques (2011): "Metamorphoses of The Uncanny In The Short-Story 'The Landlady' by Roald Dahl." In: Miranda 5, December 3, 2022 (https://www.doi.org/10.4000/miranda.2515).

Stončikaitė, Ieva (2017): "'No, My Husband Isn't Dead, [But] One Has To Re-Invent Sexuality': Reading Erica Jong For The Future of Aging." In: Societies, 7/2:11.

Stončikaitė, Ieva (2020): "To Lift or Not To Lift? The Dilemma of An Aging Face In Erica Jong's Later Works." In: Journal of Aging Studies 52.

Van Haegenborgh, Elisabeth (2015): "The Gothic In Narratives by E.A. Poe, H.P. Lovecraft and Roald Dahl." In: MA Thesis, Gent University.

Walz, Thomas (2002): "Crones, Dirty Old Men, Sexy Seniors: Representations of The Sexuality of Older Persons." In: Journal of Aging and Identity 7, pp. 99–112.

Warren, Alan (1988): Roald Dahl (Starmont Contemporary Writers), Starmont: Mercer Island.

West, Mark Irwin (1990): "The Grotesque and The Taboo In Roald Dahl's Humorous Writings For Children." In: Children's Literature Association Quarterly 15/3, pp. 115–116.

West, Mark Irwin (1992): Roald Dahl (Twayne's English Authors Series), New York: Maxwell Macmillan.

Woodward, M. Kathleen (1991): Aging And Its Discontents: Freud and Other Fictions, Bloomington: Indiana University Press.

Zeilig, Hannah (2011): "The Critical Use of Narrative and Literature In Gerontology." In: International Journal of Ageing and Later Life 6/2, pp. 7–37.

Two Witches at the School
Aging and Instruction in Argento's and Guadagnino's *Suspiria* Films

André Assis Almeida and João Paulo Guimarães[1]

> Suzy Bannion decided to perfect her ballet studies in the most famous school of dance in Europe. She chose the celebrated academy of Freiburg. One day, at nine in the morning, she left Kennedy airport, New York, and arrived in Germany at 10:40 p.m. local time.
> – Opening voiceover of Suspiria
> ... narrated in the Italian version by an uncredited Dario Argento

Pulp filmmaker Dario Argento and his then partner (and screenwriter for the project) Daria Nicolodi famously drew upon an essay by Thomas De Quincey to sketch the idea for their 1977 horror classic *Suspiria*. The piece in question integrates De Quincey's collection *Suspiria de Profundis* and is titled "Levana and Our Ladies of Sorrow". In it, the English author delves into the topic of education; not of the formal kind we get in school, but that which we acquire by way of experience. Experiences that end in grief are, according to De Quincey, particularly instructive and,

---

1   University of Porto.

albeit painful, allow a person to grow. If, from an archetypal perspective, the three Furies are the figures responsible for meting out justice and the three Muses have the roles of energizing our creative endeavors, then Levana (the Roman goddess of childbirth) and the three sisters she communes with, creations of De Quincey, the titular Ladies of Sorrow (impersonations of "the powers that shake man's heart") (De Quincey 2003:154), are in charge of our worldly edification. De Quincey gives each sister a distinct personality, thus suggesting that grief can be dealt with in different ways. So, while the Mother of Tears, the eldest of the three, symbolizes overt lamentation, the Mother of Sighs represents quiet resignation, and, lastly, the Mother of Darkness is the patron of lunacy and suicide.

> [']These are the Sorrows, all three of whom I know.' The last words I say *now*; but in Oxford I said – 'one of whom I know, and the others too surely I *shall* know.' For already, in my fervent youth, I saw ... the imperfect lineaments of the awful sisters. (De Quincey 2003: 155)

The film trilogy that Argento built around this mythos – *Suspiria*, *Inferno* and *Mother of Tears* – sees his main characters confront each of the sisters, whom he has turned into witches, to prevent them from corrupting and dominating the world, which, according to the expository narration that opens *Inferno*, is their malevolent plan. That is: the overarching symbolic implications of De Quincey's original Ladies, so essential to the essay's overall structure and meaning, are completely discarded by Argento in his films, in favor or something much more literal-minded and campy (they are now just evil witches wreaking havoc, causing death and destruction in major European and North-American towns).

This departure is obviously not a surprise, since Argento, then already known for his stylishly over-the-top *giallo* thrillers (*The Bird with the Crystal Plumage*, *The Cat o' Nine Tails*, *Deep Red*), was not the director one would expect a faithful adaptation of De Quincey from, no matter how feverish or oneiric the original material is. In fact, as Alexandra Heller-Nicholas points out in her book on *Suspiria*, "Levana and Our Lady of Sorrows" was actually a late comer to Argento's 1977 witchcraft project, arriving only after several other references and ideas were solidly in place. And, to be honest, the names in "Levana" and their sonority do seem to be the only elements that truly survive from text to screen: be it in the title of the film (taken from the whole book and not from the essay directly relating to it), or in the names of the three sisters/mothers, which, particularly in their Latin incarnations, evoke almost by themselves an ancient, eerie atmosphere – *Mater Suspiriorum*, *Mater Tenebrarum*, and *Mater Lachrymarum*. However, despite all these reservations and disconnections, there is at least one thematic concern that clearly links De Quincey's essay to Argento's *Suspiria*, and even to Guadagnino's 2018 remake of it: the preoccupation with learning. Both versions of *Suspiria* take place within school environments, a German dance academy that teaches classical ballet in the first film and modern dance in the second, and have as their main source of conflict/horror an opposition between the youthful students and their menacing instructors, who continue to be teachers even if they are also revealed to be witches. One could argue that the films work like streamlined *Bildungsromans*, telling the coming-of-age journey of our protagonist, Suzy Bannion, from childish (or late teenage) innocence to a state of maturity. Argento and Guadagnino, much like one of the seven Harry Potter novels, seem to directly associate graduating a school year with getting ready for (a sort of) adulthood. And to them, as to De Quincey, but now through horror trappings, this process of growing up can apparently only be achieved via rituals of suffering, violence, and even death.

However, learning by trauma is not a notion that is exclusive to De Quincey; and, in the sense of it being an inspiration to Argento, a more apt predecessor can surely be traced to several popular fairy tales (or fairy tale inspired works, such as *The Wizard of Oz* and *Alice in Wonderland*), which also thematize this idea. Argento, in contrast to the way he used/dismissed De Quincey, this time actively incorporated these other influences into *Suspiria*'s narrative and aesthetic aspects, constantly referencing fairy tale logic, imagery and even specific stories.

Three quick examples:

a) Without a doubt, the most consistently discussed reference to *Suspiria* is Walt Disney's 1937 animated version of *Snow White*, "which Argento has stated on numerous occasions was a direct influence on the film" (Heller-Nicholas 2015: 30). Its influence can be seen on the color palette, in the overall décor, in Argento's choice of actress Jessica Harper for lead – "I thought she would be perfect for the role of Snow White", he explains in a documentary on the 25th anniversary of *Suspiria* – and notably in the character of the ultimate witch, Helena Markos, who, similar to the Queen in *Snow White*, appears in the conclusion of the film as the typical decrepit old hag with a cartoonishly evil laughter.

b) *Suspiria*'s doors, as in *Bluebeard* and Carroll's *Alice in Wonderland*, are central to the story it tells, often acting as literal passages to fantastic worlds and/or disturbing realizations. In the first scene of the film, the unmotivated attention that Argento gives to an automated door at the airport – the jarring interruption of the soundtrack, the extreme close-up of its greasy gears, the aggressively fast sliding motion of the glass panels – already indicates to us the significance of this motif. The Freiburg dance academy itself can very well be seen as a series of locked/forbidden rooms which Suzy, in her quest to uncover the mystery of the place, must progressively open throughout the film.

c) From *Hansel and Gretel*, another important reference to *Suspiria*, at least two strong echoes can be found. First, in the bright red building of the dance academy, which, despite being a faithful recreation of a real setting, gives us a strong artificial impression, bringing to mind the alluring cake house (she wants to attract kids) of the cannibal witch from the Grimms fairy tale – the building almost looks like it could be bitten into. And second, in the climactic sequence of the film. when Suzy retraces the footsteps of the teachers, finally discovering the hidden location of the witches' coven. As has been noted by several critics, this entire plot point can be easily related to the breadcrumbs and flintstones that Hansel and Gretel use to find (and also lose) their way back home.

Guadagnino's 2018 *Suspiria* takes a markedly different approach to this matter, even appearing to harbor some sort of aversion to the kinship with fairy tales that the first film has. Moments that are objectively repeated, such as Suzy finding a hidden door and retracing footsteps, are so heavily dehydrated from this connection that they don't even register as fantastic or otherworldly. The feeling is completely different. 2018's Suzy, in a kind of a trance, simply finds a hidden door on the wall and then arrives at the lower levels of the school, where the witches are performing some kind of weird, pagan ritual.

This distancing intention is also apparent through some of the statements that the screenwriter, David Kajganich, made on the making of the film:

> And so, I said to Luca [Guadagnino] when he asked me would I ever be interested in joining him in this ... 'I will take quite a practical approach if you're okay with that. I would want to know how something like this could happen, how it would work, what the hierarchy of the coven would be, you know, all of those practical questions that normally aren't maybe of interest to a typical horror film, whatever that is,' and he was all for it. And so, I did quite a lot of research and to actual witchcraft and covens and we did quite a lot of research into the period that it's set in, what was going on in feminist politics and feminist art then, and how were concerns being exploited from the inside out and how that might look inside of the context of the occult. (Kajganich 2018)

In another interview, Kajganich says that one of his methods for constructing the film was to apply "a lot of practicality to it": grounding several elements that were only indicated or superficially treated in Argento's original (such as the cultural and political context of the setting: Germany 1977), and removing the ones "that didn't make literal sense to me" (he explicitly refers the scene where a character falls into a room filled with barbed wires). This points us to a clear divide between the two *Suspirias*, particularly in the way they choose to approach the codes and conventions of the genres they inhabit, i.e., horror and fantasy.

Argento, for example, is a filmmaker who doesn't shy away from genre clichés. Much the opposite, as noted by Marcia Landy in her study on the director, his films purposefully embrace clichés into their dramatic conceptions (2016: 106), making them a fundamental part of his kitsch, self-conscious and highly stylized approach to the medium, which often relies on a fusion of commonplace tropes (the black gloved killers, young attractive women as perpetual victims, comedic meet-cutes, cheap whodunits, etc.) and operatic exaggeration.

In *Suspiria*, therefore, Argento was also not trying to break the mold of the supernatural witchcraft film. The subversion that de facto exists within the film does not stem from Argento's rejection of the subgenre's form, but from a hyper-fetishization (in the Freudian sense of the term) of it. It's as if he had a volume dial that he cranked up to the extreme in all the elements that captivated him – such as the violence, the music, the Technicolor –, while simultaneously dialing down, almost to mute, the parts that bored him – psychological characterization, plot logic, the need for justifications. This mix of an excessive, brutish style with bare and extremely naïf elements, and the fact that this blend somehow works (which is not always the case with Argento), is to a large extent what makes *Suspiria*, event today, such a provocative and difficult to interpret project. It is a film "heavily loaded towards the senses," that combines the rejection of expected narrative paradigms "with an aggressive stylistic hyperactivity, making *Suspiria* a film that needs to be experienced through the body as much as through the intellect" (Heller-Nicholas 2015: 7). To use the film's own words, the story *Suspiria* tells (or the manner it tells it) "seems so absurd, so fantastic" that it almost does not make sense. Whereas Argento's *Suspiria* happily inhabits its horror and fantasy genre traditions, even some of the outdated ones (the maniacal cackling of the old witch, the deformed Igor-like servant, the moldy gothic-looking attic), Guadagnino's *Suspiria* is corrective to the core.

The screenplay solemnly begins with a quotation by Joseph Goebbels: "dance must be cheerful and show beautiful female bodies and have nothing to do with philosophy". The film, obviously not wanting to agree with Adolf Hitler's propaganda minister, will forcibly go in the other direction. 2018's *Suspiria* carries its critical intentions on its sleeve. The Goebbels quote is even responded to by the character of Madame Blanc, who, different from Argento's film, where all witches are simply unified evil, is on the good side of the story, being the representative of the militant side of the dance academy/witches coven. She explains to her students, and to us: "There are two things that dance can never be again. *Beautiful* [emphasis added] and cheerful. Today we need to break the nose of every beautiful thing".

The film's focus is not so much philosophy – only if we see it in the broadest of senses -, but politics and history. *Suspiria* 2018 opens with a potentially violent protest for the release of the Baader-Meinhof (there's smoke, people chanting in "organized rage", throwing things at the police barrier); a character, Patricia, who is the first victim in both works, crosses this chaotic environment to go to her psychoanalyst and talk, in an incoherent and rambling manner, about the coven of witches she fears govern her dance academy. These two worlds (or meanings), political upheaval and witchcraft, are closely connected from the very beginning of the film. The setting of the dance academy is no longer a picturesque and isolated Freiburg (magical, fairy tale Germany), but the capital Berlin, and not any place in Berlin, but right next to the Berlin Wall. The building in the new film loses its red alluring cake-house look, and is transformed into a drab, enormous bureaucratic one: very clean, very monochromatic. The main problem of the witches is an election between two competing factions for control of the coven, the more progressive one, lead by Madame Blanc, who as we said is a positive figure in the film, and the other lead by the villain, Mother Helena Markos, who wants to bring the academy/coven to its old (Nazi German?) ways.

The three characters that Tilda Swinton plays – Josef Klemperer, Mother Helena Markos, and Madame Blanc – also points us to this historical perspective:

a) Josef Klemperer, a Jewish psychoanalyst, victim of the Holocaust, who lost his wife (played by Jessica Harper, 1977 *Suspiria*'s Suzy Bannion) in the concentration camps...

b) Mother Helena Markos, a rotting, repulsive, tumor-filled and almost disabled figure, with evident Nazi ties (she even has those dark Nazi-looking aviator glasses, resembling a more deformed and less funny version of Dr. Strangelove)...

c) Madame Blanc, a more progressive witch, even if suspect at first, who feels guilt over her past actions, is critical of Germany's history, and is trying to change the coven from inside...

This triangular impasse is solved by *Suspiria* through the story-arc of Suzy Bannion. In the end, once she discovers that *she* is the actual reincarnation of *Mater Suspiriorum* – therefore, a witch herself, and the more powerful and wise of all the witches – Suzy consoles Josef Klemperer, offering him the truth about his wife's demise and allowing him to finally work through his grief; dispatches without mercy Mother Markos and all her followers ("Death to any other Mother!"); and imposes Madame Blanc's faction as the dominant one of the coven, responsible for its reconstruction. Suzy becomes the literal manifestation of a well-intentioned *Zeitgeist* of renewal, even summoning a spirit (so, a *Geist*) to do her bidding: exploding the heads of the witches who voted for Nazi Helena Marco.

The learning that Suzy Bannion does throughout *Suspiria* 2018 is both historical and political, although quite basic in the two instances: she essentially learns that Nazism was bad, still lurks in contemporary society, and must be fought against. The film then, despite all its gourmet art-house packaging and seriousness of themes (motherhood, national guilt, alternatives to patriarchal society), ends up nonetheless a rather didactic enterprise. And since didactic is not necessarily a bad adjective, let's be clear – didactic in the worst sense of the word: moralistic, superficial and heavily message-oriented.

A more instructive approach, in De Quincey's sense of the word, would have mobilized the figure of the aged witch in a more productive manner, as a symbol of death and of the inevitability of time's passing, rather than as an enemy that must be dethroned in the name of beauty, sexual liberation and youth. As Robert Graves's *The White Goddess* makes plain, the archetypal figure of the young woman as an icon of vitality is inseparable from that of the crone, harbinger of castration, barrenness and death[2]. This primal witch figure is key to a cyclical understanding

---

2   Manuela Lopez Ramirez notes that, over time, the figure of the crone, so important for the feminine holy trinity of pre-patriarchal societies, was cut off

of time according to which older age is a natural stage of life. This does not, of course, mean that the witch is unambiguously a friend, which is why the showdown between Suzie Bannion and Mother Suspiriorum, in Argento's *Suspiria*, makes dramatic sense. As much as one would like to see some sort of intergenerational reconciliation between the figures of the older woman and the young girl (which would have made the film politically progressive), it is understandable that Argento opts for a fairytale-like struggle between old age and youth.

Guadagnino handles this conflict in a way that is at first blush more empowering but in fact turns out to be somewhat problematic and perhaps even regressive. The film ostensibly puts a positive spin on the conventional image of the witch, but it in effect promotes a rather conformist view of what an autonomous, progressive and desirable woman should be. Much like her character from the popular *50 Shades* franchise, Dakota Johnson plays a girl that, during the course of her journey of self-discovery, attains sexual liberation, freely expressing sexual desires that would traditionally have been considered perverted and/or depraved. The "good" witch Susie Bannion, represents the modern woman. She comes into her own as a witch and achieves emancipation as a woman by overthrowing the covenant of ideologically conservative witches that run the Markos Dance Academy. This adds a twist to the story of the original 1977 *Suspiria* in which Susie simply dispatches Mother Markos and runs away from the collapsing dance academy, there being no further implications to this fairy tale struggle between good and evil. In Guadagnino's film we realize at the end that Susie is the true Mother Suspiriorum, a title everyone thought belonged to Mother Markos, the old hag Susie dethrones and replaces. This intergenerational showdown is seen as a token of renewal and progress by the film. We argue, however, that by

---

from the other two, vilified and transformed into the evil hag or witch that became popular in fairy tales: "The suppression of the crone figure results in the appearance of a purely wicked archetype (the witch or the hag), such as we find in fairy tales. . . . In fairy tales, the witch, the crone who stands for values our society rejects for women, is set against the stereotypical figure of the beautiful and good fairy-tale princess" (2020: 43).

championing youth and exalting Susie as a model witch, the film reinforces the idea that old witches are evil, repulsive and inconvenient[3]. In Guadagnino's film, Susie not only defeats the witch but she replaces her, becoming the leader of the coven herself. As such, the figure of the older woman, one of the three faces of Graves's eternal goddess, is vanquished and superseded. Older age is not needed, the film tells us; not even for the kind of mythic battle dramatized in Argento's film. The only lesson Guadagnino wishes to impart is that liberal values ought to always triumph in the end, no matter the cost.

Author Bios

André Assis Almeida graduated in Cinema from the Universidade Federal de São Carlos (UFSCar) and is currently pursuing a master's degree in Literary, Cultural, and Interart Studies at the Faculdade de Letras da Universidade do Porto (FLUP), where he is developing a thesis titled "The Miscellany as Method in Camilo and Ruiz's Mysteries of Lisbon". He is also a screenwriter, his most recent work being the short films "The Strange Disappearance of Comrade Kuliakov" (2022) and "Maputo" (2024).

Joao Paulo Guimaraes holds a PhD in English from the State University of New York at Buffalo. He is currently a full-time researcher at the Margarida Losa Comparative Literature Institute of the University of Porto. He is the author of the forthcoming book *American Experimental Poetry and the New Organic Form* (Bloomsbury Studies in Critical Poetics), editor of the collection *Aging Experiments: Futures and Fantasies of Old Age* (tran-

---

3   M. Isabel Santaularia i Capdevila contends that we find many examples of witches that are portrayed positively in recent popular culture. However, she notes that characters like Buffy or Hermione Granger "are almost exclusively young" (2018: 60). The "imagining of the old witch as powerful yet benign has been underexplored in popular culture" (2018: 60), Capdevila adds.

script) and is currently preparing a manuscript about older age and contemporary American innovative poetry.

Works Cited

Capdevila, M. Isabel Santaularia (2018): "Age and Rage in Terry Pratchett's 'Witches' Novels." *European Journal of English Studies* 22.1, pp. 59–75.

de Quincey, Thomas (2003): *Confessions of an English Opium-Eater and Other Writings*, London: Penguin.

Navarro, Megan (2018): "Actress Jessica Harper and Writer David Kajganich Cast Spells in 'Suspiria'. In *BloodyDisgusting* https://web.archive.org/web/20181020011810/https://bloody-disgusting.com/interviews/3524474/interview-actress-jessica-harper-writer-david-kajganich-cast-spells-suspiria/

Hagen, Kate (2018): "The Black List Interview: David Kajganich on SUSPIRIA." In *The Black List Blog*. https://blog.blcklst.com /the-black-list-interview-david-kajganich-on-suspiria-992499211bae

Heller-Nicholas, Alexandra (2015): *Suspiria*. Liverpool: Liverpool University Press.

Landy, Marcia. (2016): "The Argento Syndrome: Aesthetics of Horror." In Stefano Baschiera and Russ Hunter (eds), *Italian Horror Cinema*, Edinburgh: Edinburgh University Press.

Ramirez, Manuela Lopez (2020): "The New Witch in Toni Morrison's *Song of Solomon* and *God Help the Child*." *African American Review* 53.1, pp. 41–54.

Alzheimer's Disease as Demonic Possession in Adam Robitel's *The Taking of Deborah Logan* (2014)

Elisabete Lopes[1]

> As memories are taken one by one, it soon becomes clear that you can't run from Alzheimer's. You can only face it head-on, hopefully with dignity and hope. (*The Taking of Deborah Logan*)

Adam Robitel's *The Taking of Deborah Logan* (2014) is a horror film which documents the story of Deborah Logan (Jill Larson), a woman who is in an early stage of Alzheimer's disease. Mrs. Logan lives with her daughter, Sarah (Anne Ramsey), who is her full time caregiver. Due to the fact that they need financial aid, they both agree to participate in an academic study about mental disease carried out by a PhD student, Mia (Michelle Ang), who, together with her audiovisual crew, goes to live with the family in order to record the daily life of Mrs. Logan.

The originality of Robitel's film stems from how he resorts to the theme of possession to frame the symptoms of Alzheimer's disease such as progressive memory loss and gradual deterioration of the capacity to control bodily basic functions, something that is quite innovative

---

[1] University of Lisbon.

when it comes to horror cinema. It is along these lines that this essay aims to examine both the impact and the implications of the appropriation of a severe brain disease like Alzheimer's in the context of horror cinema. Cinema has the power to approach cultural and social issues in metaphorical ways and Robitel's work follows this trend when he ventures into the medical field to tackle the controversial subject of demonic possession.

In truth, contemporary horror cinema has shown concern for the portrayal of older people affected by degenerative illnesses (M. Night Shyamalan's *The Visit* or more recently Natalie Erika James's *Relic*). These cinematic narratives tap into two of the harrowing fears that haunt humanity: the fear of getting old and of losing both agency and identity.

As the title of the Robitel's film aptly suggests, the viewer watches Deborah Logan being "taken away", thus becoming increasingly divested of her original identity and personality by some force – disease or demonic possession – meaning that the person Deborah used to be is gradually replaced by someone (or something) that is different and displays an unusual type of behavior. In this respect, Sean Moreland (2017) acknowledges a clear affinity between the filmic register that deals with mental disorder and that which focus on demonic possession:

> Whether they treat possession as a metaphorization of mental illness, or use the phenomenological characteristics of certain mental illnesses as poetic devices for conveying the horror and anxiety of possession, each of these films draws (or attempts to draw) affective power from common anxieties about the loss of self-control and self-identity, and this should be considered as a continuum of filmic possession narratives. (Moreland 2017: 47–48)

At the beginning of the film, the spectator is provided with a portrait of a Deborah Logan who appears well groomed and elegantly dressed, cleaning the fields near her manor, in the company of her neighbor, Harry (Ryan Cutrona). When the filming crew arrives, led by Mia, a medical student, she receives them warmly, while enthusiastically announcing to her male friend Harry that "They're going to do a film about [her]"

(*The Taking of Deborah Logan*). Indeed, at first glance, there seems to be nothing wrong with that nice lady busy with her garden. As far as the group of students is concerned, she comes across as a healthy lady. However, Deborah's initial enthusiasm suddenly vanishes as, minutes later, she changes her mind, telling her daughter that she is not interested in taking part in the documentary that the university students are making about Alzheimer's disease. Sarah tells her that they really need the money to keep the manor and the property. Ultimately, Deborah acquiesces and a week later the recording sessions begin.

With the aim of conveying a faithful portrait of the daily routines of Deborah Logan, the film director resorts to the cinematic technique called "found footage". This type of cinematic register suggests a reality that although fictional, feels like something real to the spectator, as it is presented through the form of a documentary. Claudio Zanini, in "Evil and the Subversion of Factual Discourse in Found Footage Films", holds the opinion that "The appeal of found footage films derives from their *referentiality* and *evidentiality*, that is, making a reference to a fact and proving it actually happened" (2019: 32). The author likewise claims that "Like other types of false documentaries, found footage is a fictional format that presents itself in the form of non-fiction" (17). The fact that *The Taking of Deborah Logan* is recorded as "found footage" highly contributes to turn the events more credible and tangible, hence giving the viewer the impression that the horror that is afflicting that family is something that actually could be true. In this regard, Maddi McGillvray adds, "The film begins by mimicking a medical documentary through a montage of supporting documents, medical charts, and seemingly 'real' hospital footage outlining the side effects and facts about Alzheimer's disease" (McGillvray 2019:75). In these terms, horror, the traditional field of the "uncanny," becomes a more familiar territory that, by means of "found footage", is transformed into something quite homely.

Presenting the spectator with a supposedly true documentary, Robitel tries to call attention to the suffering of a woman, Deborah, who not so long ago was in the possession of her intellectual capabilities and now, due to the effects of Alzheimer's disease, is suffering from memory loss, slowly losing her sense of identity and the capacity of spatial orientation as well. To thoroughly document Deborah's routine, the crew installs cameras in several parts of the house. In the introduction to her documentary, Mia refers to Alzheimer's disease in a credible way, calling the viewers' attention both to the seriousness of the ailment and the role of the caregivers, thus highlighting that "The story of Alzheimer's is never about one person. My PhD thesis film posits that this insidious disease not only destroys the patient but also has a physiological influence on the primary caregiver" (*The Taking of Deborah Logan*). Addressing the audience, she proceeds, by providing a scientific account of the disease:

> Alzheimer's occurs when abnormal protein fragments accumulate in the hippocampus, killing neurons. The disease then creeps towards the front of the brain, wiping out neurons responsible for logical thought and problem-solving. It then assaults the sensory region, sparking terrifying hallucinations. Eventually, it erases a person's oldest and most precious memories. In the end stage, Alzheimer's destroys the part of the brain that regulates the heart and breathing. When swallowing goes, death is not far behind. (*The Taking of Deborah Logan*)

The language employed to depict the surge and escalation of the disease aptly ties in with the horror story that is about to unfold, as the disease appears as some type of evil which creeps, assaults, erases and destroys, thus culminating in the demise of the debilitated patient. These remarks pave the way for Deborah Logan's nightmare.

In order to accomplish a solid documentary, Mia starts by interviewing Deborah. Underlying this inquisitive look upon Sarah's mother lies the intention of conveying the image of a normal woman, who, despite the threat of an impending degenerative disease, still attempts to maintain the independence and autonomy that she once had. Owing to the fact that she lost her husband while she was still raising Sarah, she became a switchboard operator, having a phone station installed at her home.[2] Working from home, she could take care of her child, manage her domestic chores, as well as pursue an active lifestyle.

Throughout the film, Alzheimer's disease is not portrayed in derogatory terms, as the university crew tries to support the contents of the documentary resorting to medical evidence and providing it with a scientific background, in an attempt to somehow "normalize" Deborah's delicate health condition. As Mia narrates, "Deborah's brain is much like the switchboard she so adeptly worked on for decades [...] her misfiring synapses like the phone lines being pulled from their jacks, losing connections" (*The Taking of Deborah Logan*). This comparison plays an important role in the film, because, as Deborah herself remarks, she used to be "the nexus" (*The Taking of Deborah Logan*) of the town, that is to say, by being a professional switchboard operator, she managed to establish connections between people and process a lot of varied information. Ironically, she operated as a sort of brain, establishing the communication (neural connections) between the dwellers in Exuma.

The fear of aging that torments the majority of women is strongly addressed in Robitel's film. In more than one scene, the viewer perceives Deborah scrutinizing her image in mirror-like surfaces. This behaviour points to a double loss: on the one hand, she seems to be looking for distant memories that refuse to come back to her mind, while on the other hand, she also seems to be searching for her long-lost youth. Deep inside, Deborah seems to be looking for herself, her identity. The fact that sometimes she is seen quite agitated and wandering about the home is also a projection of this imbalance she feels growing inside of her, this phantom of forgetfulness that persists on haunting her. In this sense, she appears really disturbed by the loss of some memories that, in the past, had really been meaningful to her. For example, in a scene in which

---

2 Given her past as a switchboard operator, it is important to emphasize the importance of Deborah Logan as an intermediary in terms of the communication process. She comes across as a "channel", an image that equates her with permeability and, later on the film, provides sustenance for the emerging phenomenon of possession.

she is talking about her bedroom decoration, she forgets that she had been to Germany and that she had brought some souvenirs with her.

In an interview she gives to the university researchers, she informs them that she tries to engage herself in many activities as possible in order to slow down the disease's progression. She mentions doing puzzles and physical exercise, activities that, according to the medical expertise, will help stave off the disease. She ends the interview with a kind of hopeless remark, as she tells them: "Stave if off. There is no cure" (*The Taking of Deborah Logan*).

Actually, in one particular scene, we see Deborah nailing the windows as if wanting to stop something from getting into her house. For Sarah and the crew, this tempestive attitude means that she is increasingly becoming emotional and psychologically imbalanced. However, from a symbolical point of view, this attempt at shutting the windows permanently seems to point towards the desire of postponing the disease or keeping it at bay, thus refusing its access to both her body and mind.

In another scene, Deborah is seen disoriented, in the kitchen, desperately looking for her gardening spate. She furiously accuses the members of the crew of stealing it and, in the end, has a hysterical fit, thus becoming aggressive towards the members of the filming crew. This disturbing episode will be one of the first clues liable to signal Deborah's descent into the most severe stages of the disease.

In the beginning of the film, the spectator is informed of the intimate relationship that Deborah nurtures toward nature. She is filmed while she tends to her garden or when she is swiping off the old leaves of the manor's yard. These images seem to reiterate the symbolic feminine bond with nature and its natural cycles. Later on the film, this natural connection is gradually replaced by the medical and scientific context imposed by the severity of Deborah's mental health.

Elizabeth Bronfen, in *Over her Dead Body: Death, Femininity and the Aesthetic* (1992), highlights this bond women share with nature and the consequences of this ontological connection. As the author remarks, nature, much like women, frequently appears associated with unruly disorder and uncivilized wilderness (66), construed as Other in opposition to culture. The author observes that in the vulnerable position as the Other, woman is positioned as "object of intense scrutiny to be explored, dissected" (*Ibidem*), terms that are reminiscent of medical procedures.

While the audience accompanies the crew as they become familiarized with her routines, it learns that one of Deborah's pastimes is painting. She enjoys painting the woods surrounding her house, which, as previously mentioned, ties the feminine with the natural landscape. In her beautiful, but eerie creations, there is a pervasive shadow that, in the most recent paintings, seems to be getting bigger and closer. This shadow not only epitomizes Deborah's Alzheimer's disease, but also the upcoming phenomenon of demonic possession that she is about to encounter. One of the manifestations of possession occurs when Deborah develops a strange rash in the neck, that threatens to expand itself to her whole body. This dermatologic problem evokes the image of a snake shedding off its skin, a medical episode that can metaphorically be read as a metamorphosis. Given the circumstances, Sarah and Mia decide that it is better to take Deborah to the hospital, where she will be given medical attention. After having observed Sarah's mother, Dr. Nazir (Anne Bedian) tells them that skin problems are not usually related to the Alzheimer's disease and, as a result, Deborah is discharged from the hospital.

In another scene, that focuses upon another one of Deborah's nighttime wanderings, the crew finds her in the attic, alienated and naked, trying to use the old switchboard station.[3] She then starts to speak French in a voice that does not resemble her own. When she sees the crew, she starts unplugging cables from the station and, as a consequence, a short circuit occurs. Before the image of the camera completely fades off for some moments, the audience is able to discern the horrible figure of a monstrous man whose open mouth displays scary protruding teeth. This phantasmagorial apparition assumes the shape of a subliminal image, typical of those which intrude in horror

---

3   The scene in which Deborah is trying to use the old switchboard is highly reminiscent of the Victorian madwoman who, due to her mental problems, was confined to the attic.

films, such as William Friedkin's *The Exorcist* (1973). While analysing the recorded episode, on the crew's computer, they find out that Deborah was trying to reach the number 337 that belonged to someone named Henry Desjardins, a fact that would explain her use of the French language. Sarah informs Mia that Desjardins is quite known in Exuma, since he was an infamous serial killer who killed four children in the 1970s. Sarah tells her that there is a documentary on the subject and they both decide to watch it. In the end, both women find out that Desjardins suffered from a lethal disease and wanted, by all means, to achieve immortality. Dabbling with the occult, he decided to perform a Monacan ancient ritual that required the kidnapping and killing of five girls. The girls, referred to, in the documentary as "bleeding flowers", would be killed during the time of their first menstruation and their blood would be offered to a demon as a dark trade for immortality. The documentary provides a visual gruesome description of the girls' bodies, reporting that the girls were each found with serpentine carvings on their foreheads. Some parts of their bodies were cannibalized, and traces of rattlesnake venom were found in their blood. However, the ritual was not complete because Desjardins failed to murder the fifth girl. Before he could proceed with its sinister mission, he suddenly disappeared. In the documentary, it is said that he might have gone to Quebec or even taken his own life.

Later on, Deborah starts feeling unwell and vomits earth mixed with worms, and is, once more, taken to the hospital, in distress. While at the hospital, she tries to kidnap a little girl, who is suffering from cancer. As a result, doctors are forced to restrain her to her bed. Seeing her mother's health rapidly deteriorating, Sarah decides to seek unconventional help, outside the doctors and science's sphere.[4]

In fact, when Sarah sees her mother in the hospital bed, hysterical, screaming in a voice that does not resemble hers, she confesses to Mia that "There's something else going on" (*The Taking of Deborah Logan*). At

---

4   Sarah manages to speak to a priest, but to no avail since he displays a sceptical opinion regarding the existence of a paranormal phenomenon at the origin of Deborah's health deterioration.

that moment, Sarah decides she must do something to understand the nature of these unusual episodes that verge on the paranormal, so as to help her mother.[5] Mia agrees and starts researching in order to find someone who could be able to give them some answers. Later, they manage to meet with the Professor of Anthropology, Dr. Ernest Schiffer, who was featured in the Desjardins's documentary. First, the anthropologist tries to come up with a logical explanation, dismissing the events as being the result of Deborah's obsession with the serial killer. But, in the end, he offers Sarah and Mia an alternate explanation. He claims that the weaker minds of the infirm, the old or the children, are susceptible to attract spiritual parasites, vengeful entities, seeking a fragile host to invade. Dr. Schiffer, then, tells them about the ancient ritual that took place in the caves of the mines, in the Monacan mountains, near the river Rouge.

The fact that the anthropologist speaks of possession, employing medical terminology, claiming that it is caused by a spiritual parasite, ultimately means that, like Alzheimer's, a demonic assault can also be viewed as a type of disease. Indeed, the man's words imply that Sarah's mother could be possessed by the spirit of Henry Desjardins. In fact, Desjardins himself was suffering from a degenerative disease at the time of the crimes, more precisely, he had Lou Gehrig's disease. With the aim of keeping the disease at a distance, or "stave it off" (if we choose to use Deborah's terms), he turned to black magic with the intention of performing a ritual. In the film both diseases, Alzheimer's and Lou Gehrig's disease, appear as degenerative ailments that are strongly tied in with the phenomenon demonic possession.

Later in the film, it is revealed to the viewer that Sarah was indeed the fifth girl, the one that would enable Desjardins to accomplish the last stage of the ritual. At the time, Deborah apparently became acquainted with the evil man's intentions and, together with her neighbour and

---

5   Contrasting with previous horror films that focus on demonic possession, in *The Taking of Deborah Logan*, it is the feminine partnership developed between Sarah and Mia that will gather efforts to attend to Deborah's possession, instead of a male priest or exorcist.

best friend Harry, decided to set the doctor up, hence killing him and burying him in the forest adjacent to Deborah's manor. However, this action comes with a price because the doctor's demonic spirit is later able to possess Deborah. The fact that she was a "professional communicator" turns her into the perfect shelter for a hostile spirit because, to a certain extent, she can be seen as a channel, due to her professional past as a phone worker. In the film, Mia's account echoes this thought as she states, referring to Sarah's mother, "Deborah's brain is much like the switchboard she so adeptly worked on for decades... her misfiring synapses like the phone lines being pulled from their jacks, losing connections" (*The Taking of Deborah Logan*).

In this respect, Carol J. Clover observes that, in horror films, the female body is liable of being colonized by external entities (102), due to its inherent physical and emotional openness. As the author observes, "... occult films code emotional openness as feminine, and figure those who indulge it, male and female as physically opened, penetrated. The language and the imagery of the occult film is thus necessarily a language and imagery of bodily orifices and insides (or a once removed but transparently related language of doors, gates, portals, channels, inner rooms)" (1992:101). According to Clover, then, "satanic possession is gendered feminine" (1992: 72) precisely due to the latent permeability that characterizes the female body.

Near the epilogue, the spectator sees Deborah walking through the corridors of the hospital. In one of the walls, we can glimpse the drawing of a snake, confirming that the old lady is, indeed, possessed by the spirit of the killer. The snake, a symbol for health is also transformed, in this horror narrative, into a beacon of sin since it signals the possession of Deborah Logan by the demon that was previously lodged in Desjardin's body. Ultimately, she manages to leave the hospital facilities, thus taking Cara (Julianne Taylor) a little girl suffering from cancer, with her, with the aim of coming to terms with the ritual that was left unfinished by the doctor. She then carries the child to a dark cave beneath the old mines, located in the mountains, which, in allegorical terms, is equated with a feminine space that resembles the womb. The scene in which Deborah is at the cave with Cara, hints at her intimate desire of becoming young again, of restoring her lost youth. The fact that the old woman is seen with her stretched mouth, trying to devour the girl's head, strongly evokes a wish for assimilation, of bodily fusion that verges on the abject. Deborah's fragile and emaciated body combined with her bloodied mouth, points to a dual image where the (pre) menstruated young body intersects with the menopaused old body, an image which results in an abject and monstrous depiction.

On a symbolic level, the cave configures a feminine space that metaphorically evokes the womb. Moreover, according to James Marriot, being inside the cavern or the cave, figuratively points to the risk of "being assimilated, losing one's identity, being devoured" (Marriot, 2013:40), an aspect that is clearly at stake in *The Taking of Deborah Logan*.

In the specific context of Robitel's cinematography, this uterine space of the cave is likened to the Alzheimer's disease and to demonic possession since both ailments threaten to swallow and erase Deborah's identity. In horror films that tackle feminine issues, Barbara Creed argues that such a uterine-like space signals the presence of the archaic mother, a mythical being which is never clearly seen on screen, but whose presence can be perceived through special metaphors, such as the cavern. The scene in the cave hints at the presence of the archaic mother, since that the dark, confined, and damp space summons the figure of the mother "as originating womb" (Creed, 1992:26). Creed defines the archaic mother as the "parthenogenetic mother, the mother as primordial abyss, the point of origin and the end" (Creed, 1992:17). It is pre-symbolic; it represents the negative counterpart of the nurturing mother and constitutes a pervasive reference in the horror film. Her visual presence is felt subtly and indirectly though, as it is depicted through a certain type of iconography such as dark humid underground spaces, tunnels, cobwebs, cellars, steep stairs, blood, earth.

Notably, in *The Taking of Deborah Logan*, the initial pastoral landscape conveyed by the placid image of Deborah working in her garden, comfortably embraced by the all-encompassing forest, is later replaced by a cavernous environment, a visual transformation that can be said to figuratively mirror Deborah's growing mental deterioration caused by the disease. It is precisely in the cave that Deborah physically displays her monstrousness by becoming a reptilian figure, with her mouth, tainted with blood, stretched in a gruesome and unnatural manner. Drawing on Linda Williams' seminal essay "When the Woman Looks" (1984), we can say that, by virtue of the phenomenon of possession, Deborah Logan's gaze becomes convergent with the monster's, thus paving the way for a perfect identification between both. Nevertheless, the monstrous figure can allow some space for the old female character to express herself free from constraints or taboos. In this respect, Rikke Schubart reminds us that the monster "can be seen as a dynamic site of meaning-making (...) and also as a method to enter a position of dialogue with what is outside society's norm, what is strange, foreign, 'Other'" (Schubart 2019: 195). This otherness then surfaces on screen due to Deborah's monstrous body and via Alzheimer's. It can be said that the monster and the disease both converge towards her corporeality, therefore rendering her identity uncanny. Amelia DeFalco, in *Uncanny Subjects: Aging in Contemporary Narrative* (2010) states,

> Dementia provides caregivers, storytellers, with dramatic lessons of uncanny identity. Not only is there the obvious uncanniness of the victim whose deteriorated memory produces a frightening strangeness, but there is often self-revelation for the storyteller who comes to recognize his or her own otherness in the process of collaborating with the afflicted (DeFalco 2010:59-60).

It is precisely this frightening strangeness that emanates from the vision of the altered Deborah that ultimately transforms her into a monster.[6] Fred Botting, in his seminal oeuvre *Gothic* (1992), argues that monsters "give shape...to obscure fears and anxieties, or contain an amorphous and unrepresentable threat in a single image" (Botting: 8). In fact, the fear elicited by Deborah's possession allied to the disease and its effects turn her into a monstrous figure that becomes more frightful in the

---

6 Deborah's cinematic descent into possession can indeed epitomize the current cinematic phenomenon that Elizabeth Herskovits deems the "monsterizing of senility" (Herskovits 1995:153).

sense that it turns a mirror to the audience whereby it shows the phantom of old age lurking ahead, waiting for them as a potential threat in the future.

The fact that Desjardins's ritual involved young girls about to experience their first menstruation, heavily contrasts with Deborah's old age. In a symbolic plan, we have female menopause as an omen of lack of strength and physical and mental deterioration, while the surge of menarche suggests life and the capability of reproduction and subsequent renovation. Nevertheless, in an intelligent twist, the film's director can be said to craft a subversive visual narrative, since he also endows Deborah with reproductive powers, as she is able to transmit her possession to the little girl. From an non reproductive status afforded by her biological age, Deborah becomes productive and fertile again, thus playing an active role in the transference of Desjardin's evil to the little girl.

At some point, when both Mia and Sarah are chasing Deborah through the cave system, the first woman informs the latter "Whatever this is, it is not your mom." This form of disavowal is liable to be applied to Deborah to the degree that she is victim of demonic possession, and Alzheimer's, a double threat, as both phenomena (paranormal and scientific) rob the person of their identity, leaving them divested of their personality traits. In other words, the possessed woman and the Alzheimer's patient have been robbed of their selves; they are turned into mere vessels. Both body and mind reflect that "lesser status" of a person who is on the verge of losing full autonomy and whose memories are liable to become fractured and unreliable. In this regard, Deborah can be said to face a double battle, as possession also involves dispossession, to the extent that her memories and identity are held hostage to an entity or degenerative disease.[7]

---

7   A fundamental difference between traditional films which tackle possession and Robitel's film is that in the former, symptoms of the demonic possession are read as if they were a disease whereas in *The Taking of Deborah Logan* this logic is reversed: Deborah's disease degenerates into a possession case.

In a more benign perspective, this alliance between demonic possession and the Alzheimer's disease can be said to forge the phenomenon of 'transaging' that conveys a fluid image concerning the perception of the aging process. In "Un/re/production of Old Age in *The Taking of Deborah Logan*" (2018), Agnieszka Kotwasińska, appropriates Helen Moglen's concept of transaging and adapts it to Deborah Logan's peculiar situation. According to Moglen, transaging encapsulates "the constant, erratic movement that takes place in consciousness across, between and among the endlessly overlapping stages of life" (Chen & Moglen 2006:139). It consists of a dynamic concept which entails aging as something fluid and not compartmentalized into stages. Deborah Logan, due to the effects provoked by Alzheimer's disease, loses herself in her memories and is able to inhabit both the past and the present simultaneously. In this way, Kotwasińska contends that the phenomenon of possession makes possible the co-existence of different personas such as the single mother, the businesswoman, the murderess and the elderly lady that form part of Deborah's self. In the author's viewpoint, the several identities "are not temporarily disengaged from each other but form one vibrant mesh that Deborah experiences simultaneously through her body memory" (Kotwasińska 2018:188). Indeed, in Deborah's case, bodily memory prevails over the vulnerable cognitive memory, a reality that heavily contributes to render Deborah's body a place of meaning. As Magrit Shildrick contends, "The body [...] is not a prediscursive reality, but rather a locus of production, the site of contested meanings, and as such fluid and unstable, never given and fixed" (Shildrick 2002:10). In Robitel's film, Deborah's body comes across as a site of inscription and revisitation of selves that co-habit her simultaneously forming a fluid path between the past, the present and the future.

In the end, the young girl is saved by Sarah, who is forced to shoot her mother in order to stop her nefarious action.

Following the ordeal involving the kidnapping of the child by Deborah, the journalists announce in the media that the girl was able to mysteriously fight the cancer that was consuming her. Hungry for a sensationalist story, they interview her while she is celebrating her birthday. She seems happy now that she is fully recovered. When the journalist asks her what her plans to the future are, she enigmatically says that she has some, but she cannot reveal them yet, an announcement that leaves the audience guessing that the child might be possessed by Desjardins's spirit.

While Cara meets a joyful destiny, as she is restored to the family safe and sound, Deborah, in turn, is shown heavily debilitated, being escorted in a wheelchair by her daughter. Her semblant reveals alienation and absence. In truth, she is portrayed as if she were a vacant body, now totally dependent on her daughter. This elicits a sense of horror that has a double effect: on the one hand Cara is healed, but possessed; on the other, Deborah physical and mental decay seem to have taken root.

Moreover, this final image that the film conveys of Deborah, of a frail body absent of soul, is evocative of the cinematic zombie, an image which resonates with some scientific articles that, when dealing with health issues, such as dementia and the Alzheimer's disease, tend to compare the Alzheimer's patient to a zombie, someone "whose brain has been destroyed by the disease and who therefore no longer exists as a person but only as a body to be managed" (Behuniak 2011: 74), meaning a real walking dead. In this context, Susan M. Behuniak argues that the fictional character of the zombie has "leaked into the popular and scholarly discourse about real people who have Alzheimer's disease, constructing them as animated corpses and their disease as a terrifying threat to the social order" (Behuniak 2011: 72). Sharing the same perspective, Gerry Canavan also believes the zombie is lately being treated, in cinematic terms, as "an allegory for the disabled or infirm body, particularly, the elderly body" (Canavan 2016:17).

Apart from evoking the zombie,[8] Deborah becomes the physical repository for several iconographic characters from horror films as her personal story progresses. She can be said to epitomize the figure of the vampire, especially in the scene where we see her in the cave about

---

8   Following the scene in which Deborah is found in the attic, undressed, and tampering with her old switchboard, she has a fit and consequently vomits a black liquid substance in which mud is mixed with earthworms, an image that evokes the figure of the zombie or a dead body.

to attack the little girl, in which she appears impossibly pale with a bloodied mouth. She can also be said to invoke the character of the evil witch who, in the majority of fairy tales abducts children so as to cause them harm. Another mythical figure of horror that is summoned in the film is the Medusa. Indeed, when Deborah is taken to the hospital, we see her laid on the bed, with her hair spread upon the pillow, strongly suggesting the iconography of the frightening Medusa, whose look can kill. The emergence of this frightful iconography intrinsically suggests something which is much more horrible than being petrified. It has implicit the metamorphosis of a living subject into an objectified condition. In sum, it offers the onlookers the view of what it is like to be alive in a death-like state. Within this context it is important to underline the fact that Desjardins used snake-related imagery in his occult practices, a twofold symbol that both stands for health and the demonic.

By intermingling a degenerative disease with the supernatural phenomenon of demonic possession, Robitel tries to convey a vivid image of what it is like to experience a living nightmare. Throughout the cinematic depiction of Deborah's nightmare, Robitel builds an insightful commentary on the impact of a serious degenerative disease, like Alzheimer's, upon the patient and the caregiver, creatively refashioning it as a demonic possession.

Indeed, memory works as a repository of individual experience that strongly contributes to forming one's personality. The usurpation of someone's past experience, whether by means of disease or by means of possession, appears as something highly threatening to human integrity and configures an uncanny experience for the caregivers as well. As Erin Harrington (2021) contends, horror films, "offer a carnivalesque space in which to act 'inappropriately', but they also centralize the importance of women, their experiences, their fears and their relationships at the center of the story" (255). By aptly weaving the threads of the natural with those of the supernatural, *The Taking of Deborah Logan* reinforces this feeling that the patient must fight to delay the disease, that ultimately means the dis-possession of identity.

Author Bio

Elisabete Lopes is an English Professor at the Polytechnic Institute of Setúbal, and a Researcher at the ULICES (Centre for English Studies of the University of Lisbon). She holds a Master's Degree in English Studies (2003) and a PhD in North-American Literature (2013). The Gothic genre, Horror cinema/literature, and Women Studies have been privileged areas of research and publication in the course of her academic career.

Works Cited

Behuniak, Susan M. (2011), "Construction of People with Alzheimer's Disease as Zombies." In: Ageing & Society 31, Cambridge Journals, Cambridge University Press, pp. 70–92.
Botting, Fred (2014): Gothic. London and New York: Routledge.
Bronfen, Elisabeth, (1992): Over her Dead Body: Death, Femininity and the Aesthetic. Manchester: Manchester University Press.
Canavan, Gerry, (2016), "Don't Point that Gun at my Mum-Geriatric Zombies." In: Lorenzo Servitje/Sherryl Vint (eds.), The Walking Med: Zombies and the Medical Image, Pennsylvania: The Pennsylvania University Press, pp. 17–38.
Chen, Nancy N./Moglen, Helen (2006): Bodies in the Making: Transgressions and Transformations, California: New Pacific Press.
Clover, Carol J. (1992): Men, Women and Chainsaws: Gender in the Modern Horror Film. Princeton: Princeton University Press.
Creed, Barbara (1993): The Monstrous Feminine: Film, Feminism, Psychoanalysis, London and New York: Routledge.
DeFalco, Amelia (2010): Uncanny Subjects: Aging in Contemporary Narrative, Columbus: The Ohio State University Press.
Harrington, Erin, (2021): Gynaehorror: Women, Monstrosity and Horror Film, New York: Routledge.
Herskovits, Elizabeth (1995): "Struggling over Subjectivity: Debates about the 'Self' and Alzheimer's Disease." In: Medical Anthropology Quarterly, 9/2, pp. 146–164.

Hodge, Mathew/Elizabeth Kusko (2020): Exploring the Macabre, Malevolent and Mysterious: Multidisciplinary Perspectives. Cambridge: Cambridge Scholars.

Kotwasińska, Agnieszka (2018), "Un/re/production of Old Age in *The Taking of Deborah Logan*." In: Somatechnics 8/2, pp. 178–194.

Marriot, James (2013): The Descent, Liverpool, Auteur, Liverpool University Press.

McGillvray, Maddi, (2019) "'To Grandmother's House We Go': Documenting Horror of the Ageing Woman in Found Footage Films." In: Cynthia A. Miller/Bowdoin Van Riper (Eds.), Elder Horror: Essays on Film's Frightening Images of Ageing, Jefferson: McFarland and Company, pp. 70–80.

Miller, Cynthia A./Bowdoin Van Riper, eds. (2019): Elder Horror: Essays on Film's Frightening Images of Ageing, Jefferson: McFarland and Company.

Moreland, Sean, (2017), "Spirit Possession, Mental Illness, and the Movies, or What's Gotten into you?" In: Sharon Packer (ed.), *Mental illness in Popular Culture*, Denver: Praeger, pp. 45–54.

Shildrick, Margrit, (2002): Embodying the Monster: Encounters with the Vulnerable Self, London: Sage Publications.

Schubart, Rikke, (2019), "'How Lucky you are never to know what it is to grow old': Witch as Fourth-wave Monster in Contemporary Fantasy Film." In: Nordlit 42, Manufacturing Monsters, pp. 191–206.

Zanini, Claudio Vescia, "Evil and the Subversion of Factual Discourse in Found Footage Films." In: Rallie Murray/Stefanie Schnitzer (eds.) Piercing the Shroud: Destabilizations of 'Evil,' Leiden and Boston: Brill Rododpi, pp. 11–33.

Williams, Linda, (1984), "When the Woman Looks." In: Mark Jancovich, The Horror Film Reader, London: Routledge, 2001, pp. 61–66.

Beyond the Horror of the Aging Female
Decay, Regeneration and *Relic*
(Natalie Erika James, 2020)

Laura Hubner[1]

The focus of this chapter is the contemporary horror film *Relic* (the debut feature made by Japanese-Australian writer and director Natalie Erika James, in 2020). A devastatingly moving film, it confronts dementia,[2] (mental and some physical) decline, decay, and loss with original sensitivity, while still drawing on conventional horror tropes. Described as both "genuinely terrifying" and equally "heart-breaking", *Relic* stands out as a horror genre movie that is as emotionally relentless and resoundingly personal as it is "spine-tingling" (Kermode 2020). The film pivots around the elderly and widowed Edna (Robyn Nevin), mother to Kay (Emily Mortimer) and grandmother to Sam, Kay's daughter (Bella Heathcote). The opening drama is triggered as Edna goes curiously missing, bringing Kay and Sam back to the deteriorating family home, nestled in the vast woodlands of Creswick (Victoria, Australia), to look for her. When Edna inexplicably reappears a few days later, barefoot and bedraggled from a few days in the woods, she is unable to recount where she has been, leaving Kay and Sam increasingly tormented by the problem of how to deal with Edna's faltering memory, her fear of intruders and her volatile, sometimes violent, actions. However, if the

---

1 University of Winchester.
2 While not a term used directly in the movie, "dementia" is referred to in some of the film's descriptions and marketing, such as the International Movie Database (IMDB) entry https://www.imdb.com/title/tt9072352/.

focus of the problem seems to be upon Edna alone, I suggest the film's unique and complex manipulations of time and space, playing with long traditions of fairytale, gothic and abject horror, ensure that any sense of "othering" the aging female, or of "othering" Edna's aging state, is radically shattered as the forces of the decaying and morphing house (increasingly a metaphor or vision of the human condition) seep outwards to affect the next generations. Edna's condition becomes theirs and ours – in a way that is immediately refreshing for a horror film. The broad stimulus here for my chapter is *women* and aging in horror movies, which traditionally has not been at all progressive. Aging women do not generally fare well in the horror film (conveyed as ugly, evil, lecherous, and ravenous). Therefore, I will begin with a glimpse at horror cinema's predominantly problematic approaches to female aging.

Gothic texts are rife with hauntings by a crazy, and often sexually experienced or dangerous, older woman, inhabiting a remote house or locked away in the attic, othered and contained from society. Connections can be made with folkloric traditions, as Sue Matheson (2019: 85) expounds: "Generally malevolent, the hags of folklore are vicious (and often malicious) embodiments of death that represent the dissolution of the body, the destructive, devouring nature of time, and the mindless persistence of the past." Conventions of presenting women as monstrous in nature (*naturally* wild, possessed, non-human or untamed), are well-documented. Barbara Creed writes of the "monstrous feminine" of more graphic or abject horror – monstrous in relation to specifically female, reproductive functions – "the archaic mother, the monstrous womb, the witch, the vampire, and the possessed woman" (Creed 1993: 73). She suggests this is connected to a fear of the female's generative power, passing from mother to daughter, relating her to the animal world in a "great cycle of birth, decay and death" (Creed 1993: 43). In fairytale horror, the evil witch, hag or crone is synonymous with physical signs of female aging: a bent frame; a raspy cackle; wispy, unmanaged gray hair; facial whiskers and bumps that denote a manipulating, hungry or interfering character living alone in the woods, sporting a broomstick. As Lynne Segal argues, with respect to the "terrifying images" of "the hag, harridan, gorgon, witch or Medusa" that myth and folktale feed to us from birth: "Such frightening figures are not incidentally female, they are quintessentially female, seen as monstrous because of the combination of age and gender." (2014: 13)[3] This reaches back to a sense of the aging female being surplus to culture, or existing on the margins of society.[4]

I raise all this because there are hints at many of these traditions in *Relic* – sometimes no more than a knowing wink, while at other points a direct confrontation or dialogue with them. However, I suggest the film is refreshingly progressive in many ways. While not unequivocally progressive, it does shake expectations, ultimately, by encouraging contemplation, empathy (rather than difference) or self-reflection, and by avoiding some of the jump scares traditionally associated with rapid female aging and decay.

The manipulation of time has played a significant role in perpetuating traditionally disturbing female old age, where sudden female aging is the focus for the terrifying. In *The Shining* (Stanley Kubrick, 1980), for example, on entering the forbidden Room 237 and embracing his fantasy, the dream turns to nightmare for Jack Torrance (Jack Nicholson), as he witnesses the young woman (object of male fantasy) becoming horrifyingly old. He catches sight of their reflection in the bathroom mirror. It is the aging process itself, and the rapidly decomposing body, visually sped up, that is the producer of horror – the visual jump scare. As Jack quickly exits the room, she staggers forwards towards him – hands reaching out to try to catch him, as he locks her back in the room. 15 years before *The Shining*, The Hammer Film *She* (Robert Day, 1965) made rapid female aging its final jump scare. Ayesha (Ursula Andress) – who throughout the film has used the magic of the blue flame to sustain eternal youth (and power) – finds this magic reversed at the end – leaving her a tragic, but mostly repulsive, figure. The young male lover recoils in horror, as the

---

3   We might note *Whatever Happened to Baby Jane* (Robert Aldrich, 1962) as an example of the close pairing between aging woman and horror.
4   Lynne Segal (2014: 43) discusses the economic burdens traditionally associated with the folkloric witch (constituting the older woman living alone) and moreover Hollywood's punishment of female characters who have gained power through independence.

rotting corpse leans towards him and collapses to the floor. The familiar horrific transformation frequently associated with vampires, werewolves and zombies here applies to witnessing a woman growing old and decaying.

I suggest that such othering by jump-scare tactics is refuted in *Relic*. While the film does have its suspense and scares (for example uncertainties lie under the bed and behind clothes in the closet) and growing images of monstrous decomposition that take over towards the end, by conveying subjects slowly, with a brooding suspense, much of the film reaches out to provoke contemplation and empathy. The first sight of Edna in *Relic* is of her stood naked in the hallway of her home with her back to us in the dimness of the night looking towards the Christmas tree fairy lights glowing on and off in the living room. The shot is poignant rather than shocking. The pool of water at her feet subtly evokes loss, growing from the slow drip from the bathroom upstairs, in a style reminiscent of Hideo Nakata's Japanese film *Honogurai mizu no soko kara* / Dark Water (2002). It suggests perhaps she forgot to turn the taps off – something the film will return to later with the discovery of her many post-it note reminders around the large house, one reading (notably written in capitals) "TURN OFF TAP" discovered by Sam when she gets into the bath. The Christmas tree provokes a sense of foreboding, like a heart pulsating, and gains significance later when Sam finds hordes of old Christmas decorations stuffed floor to ceiling in a locked room (Christmas being a time often associated with ritual, togetherness and making memories). Thus, the scene has quite the opposite effect of the naked female in *The Shining* as Edna turns her face around to the left slightly. There is no horror in her naked body or face. The moment is slow, and contemplative – with a menacing soundtrack, and rising breaths, conveying Edna's fear.

Indeed, time is key to the slow, brooding atmosphere of horror created. When Kay and Sam first enter the house to look for Edna, a bowl of decaying fruit comes into view, caught in close-up by the itinerant camera. Most immediately, it indicates Edna's withdrawal and disappearance, but the camera's static attention to the fruit and the surrounding domestic objects, and the way the items are framed, allows for a focus on stillness and time for contemplation. In this sense, the shot functions like a *vanitas*: still-life artworks popular in the 16th and 17th centuries of symbolic objects designed to get the viewer to reflect on mortality and transience, emphasising the vanity or emptiness of earthly or individual achievements. It provides a refocusing on what is important – a theme I will return to at the end of this chapter. In terms of time, broadly speaking, much of the film's events are plausible, albeit with a continual pulsating groaning soundtrack, occasional lapses into uncertain visions (of a figure in the corner and expanding rot), and interludes of nightmare visions, provoking fear, suspense, and uncertainty. But time and space break down completely in the final 20 minutes of the film, as the house stretches and shrinks, and as the mould (or bruising) grows across the building and Edna's body.

However, even in the earlier stages, time is unsettled. The past and future echo in the present. For instance, the conversation from the past of the policeman telling Kay her mother is missing plays on the soundtrack as a voice-over when Kay and Sam drive to Edna's house, and in turn when Kay travels to be interviewed further, her future conversation with the police officer is projected onto the present via voice-over as she drives. These out-of-time devices saturate the film. The policeman's words "we need a timeline" – as he tries to piece together Edna's movements before going missing – express the search for a rational, linear explanation of life, which acts as a striking contrast to the way the film itself works. Relics of Edna's previous affluent, active life are evident in the sagging tennis court net and the shot of what seems to be an old swimming pool. Their current state of disrepair is a moving reminder of a past life we can but imagine. The stained-glass window in the front door of Edna's house is a relic from the old cabin where Kay's great grandfather lived out his days by himself on this land. When looking at Edna's old beautiful drawings of woodland, Kay finds Edna's sketches of how the windows would be removed and implanted in the new building. But Kay tells Sam that apparently the old man's "mind wasn't all there in the end", and nobody had realised how bad it was. The thought of this still plagues Kay in nightmares of her great grandfather dying alone in the cabin, his rotting body falling off the bed. As the film progresses Kay's nightmare images of her great grandfather are overtaken by similar visions of her mother. Thus, the family "curse" of past abandonment is kept alive in the relic of the stained-glass window, now embedded in the house's main door, and in the film's haunting repetition of shots of stained-glass windows.

Further to this, point-of-view and close-up shots aid the subtle shift of focus from a sense of rational explanation towards experiencing and feeling Kay's concerns first-hand. For example, a shot from Kay's viewpoint when she has spotted the armchair facing the wrong way (out to the window, rather than towards the television) helps convey her shock directly. As we later find out, her mother had phoned her saying things had moved and changed, including the armchair facing out to the window. While Kay passes this off later as her mother's own doing (saying "She's doing it – she forgets things"), it still unsettles her when she sees it. It represents an early sensation of the daughter beginning to feel the shudders directly herself. She doesn't let on to Sam. Later Kay lugs the chair back to the "right" place. An extreme close-up draws attention to the foot of the chair being returned to the deep indentation of the carpet where it stood unmoved over time. Kay is both doing this for her mother and for herself – wanting things to stay as they were, actively and very decisively returning it to how it has been.

Relic draws from and complexifies traditional fairytale relationships and spaces, focusing on the three generations of women.[5] At the start, Kay might be seen as the slightly detached working mother, who wants to move her mother to a care home in Melbourne, the city where Kay lives. Creswick is about 122 kilometres northwest of Melbourne, so a fair distance for Kay to come but driveable. But later Kay retracts from the idea, after visiting a care home, and witnessing her mother's pain, suggesting in the end she move in with her in Melbourne. Idealistic Sam on the other

---

5   Cp. "Little Red Riding Hood", for example. We might also recall that some fairy tales and myths revolve around a "triple goddess" formula of maiden, mother and crone. The seeming inevitability of this triad, or female trajectory through life, alludes to that which is passed down through the generations, but perpetuated by societal treatment.

hand initially wants to move in with her gran and take care of her but must face up to her grandmother's accidents – some of them hazardous to herself or dangerous to others (at one point for example her grandmother violently snatches back the ring she gave Sam, drawing blood and accusing her of being a thief).[6]

However, the narrative is shown to be more complex than simply the mother and daughter figures finding their own roles *in relation to* the elderly female. The film more importantly concerns Kay and Sam feeling and experiencing Edna's plight themselves, as part of a repeated cycle of the human condition. Increasingly we see the characters merge. When Sam breaks through a door to find a room stuffed with old treasures, including Christmas decorations, relics of Christmases past, that grow over time, but stored for the possibilities of those in the future, she finds a photograph of an idyllic, sunny moment of family togetherness – eating outside. The photograph captures the family unposed, unaware of the camera. Edna carries the food for the table. They are drinking fresh orange juice and wearing sun hats. Due to cinematography and reflections at play, we see three Sams: 1) the current Sam (the back of her head); 2) the (only very slightly younger) Sam in the photo – reminding us times change quickly – with her grandparents protectively huddled around behind her, and 3) the reflection of her looking at the photograph. These moments of stillness in the film allow time for contemplation, even time to wonder who took the photograph – or even if it was perhaps Kay who took it. The camera lens adjustment changes, so that Sam's face comes into full focus – leaving the image of the grandparents as a ghostly trace, and Sam's own image submerging her grandmother's.[7] It is a purely cinematic moment. The photograph evokes Roland Barthes' concept of

---

6   Incidentally, the grandmother's passing on of her wedding ring to her granddaughter Sam suggests the attempt to perpetuate age-long patriarchal traditions (Edna says that Kay – the mother – did not succeed in making "any good use" of the ring). While we know in the background that Kay's marriage did not work out, none of this plays out in the film's present.

7   A similar set up, albeit more immediately terrifying, occurs in the American film *The Visit* (M. Night Shyamalan, 2015) when the girl looks in the mirror and sees the grandmother figure behind her.

death in the photographic image, as formulated in *Camera Lucida*, as it has captured a moment, like an insect in amber, embalming time: "For the photograph's immobility is somehow the result of a perverse confusion between two concepts: the Real and the Live: by attesting that the object has been real, the photograph surreptitiously induces belief that it is alive, because of that delusion which makes us attribute the Reality an absolutely superior, somehow eternal value; but by shifting this reality to the past ('this has been'), the photograph suggests that it is already dead." (Barthes 1982: 79) In this instance, the photograph provides a glimpse of a time when Edna's husband was still alive. And the cinematography and framing observe the sense of renewal or regeneration – a carrying down through the generations. In terms of the narrative, it encourages a time of reflection, and self-insight. We might ask ourselves why we take photographs of family gatherings.

Connections like this between Sam and the grandmother are made throughout the film, as are the everyday frictions that arise between mother and daughter, and the merging of roles women experience through a lifetime. To calm the nerves when Edna is still missing, Kay starts idly having a try at playing Beethoven's "Für Elise" on the piano but keeps getting stuck, when Sam walks by saying it is D after that bit not E: "Gran taught me". Kay's response to this – "Of course she did. I could never get the curl of the fingers right... I think she gave up on me at a certain point" – conveys the frictions that are commonplace in mother and daughter relationships. Soon after this, we witness the next generation repeating itself when Sam (while eating pizza) has a go at the candle carving her gran has been occupied with, drawing attention both to the connections between grandmother and granddaughter and continuing frictions between mother and daughter. Sam's mother, from the next room where she is washing up, and having found out Sam's gallery work didn't work out, is asking whether she will return to university. The calling from one room through to the next is indicative of the continual flow of these intergenerational relationships, as Kay says: "So, what – you just going to work in a bar for the rest of your life?" and Sam replies: "Maybe." We feel the responsibilities of Kay as mother – plagued by work phone calls and emails throughout the film. But moments later, (young and old at the same time) doubting the way she is dealing with her mother's disappearance, she is reassured by Sam that she is doing the right thing. For this moment, Sam takes on the parental role to console her mother, mirroring Kay's role reversal with her own mother. Many of the shots in *Relic* are filmed from another room, peering through a door or archway, with parts of the room we are looking into obscured from view. This helps to emphasize stylistically the merging between the three generational roles. For instance, at one point Kay is talking to her mother, Edna (out of view), but we only discover later when the camera adjusts that Sam is there in the foreground too.

In the final 20 minutes of the film, as rational time and space collapse completely, Sam becomes lost in a labyrinth of extra corridors and dead ends belched out by the remains of the house, screaming to find her way out, calling her mum, and banging on walls. In moments of uncanny horror, she finds herself back where she was before, and then when searching for her, Kay also becomes embroiled in the mayhem. In the end, Sam finds a way to bash through from the other side of the house, and a chase ensues as Kay and Sam help each other back through to the main house, followed by Edna, in a grotesque form of rebirth – an acceptance of aging, death and decay. Kay and Sam thus experience directly the feelings of loss and confusion felt by Edna.

The repetitions through the generations of three women permeate the film. This is conveyed visually one evening when each in turn come to brush their teeth in front of the mirror. Sam initially joins Kay, then Edna appears in the adjoining mirror. The close-ups on the reflections of each face simultaneously unite and separate the three figures, reminding us of their integral connection with each other, their impermeable similarity, as well as the pain of their being at crucially different stages of life – with time dividing but inevitably joining them. We are made aware of the interchangeable relationships from the film's start with the echoing of calls "Mum" and "Gran" when Kay and Sam first arrive. Edna confuses the names Kay and Sam several times, but we as viewers get confused too – more than once there seems to be the uncanny sense initially that it is Edna (on the stairs, or in the bath) and it turns out to be Sam. Many times, there is a confusion over which of the three is pictured lying in bed. Despite the different forms of light source each of the three women use to find their way in the darkness – a candle, a torch and a mobile phone – the *repetition* of the action (of needing to light the way) is also striking.

To explore the sense of "the Uncanny" in more depth, it is worth examining the gothic tonal qualities that surround Edna's home from the earliest stages of the film. The large haunted, possessed, or crumbling house is a staple setting for gothic literature and film, which – via transgressive possibilities and stylistic excesses – articulates the haunting return of the past seeping through the crevices into the present, or the notion that horror upsurges from within – shattering boundaries between then and now, the self and "other", internal and external or rigid concepts of "home". Sigmund Freud's essay "The Uncanny" (2003 123–162), originally published in 1919, is valuable for considering tensions between "public" and "private", or external and internal, that are central to gothic. Freud (2003: 126–134) investigates the German root of "uncanny" / "*unheimlich*" (unhomely, unfamiliar) all the way to its opposite "*heimlich*". It helps understand how the uncanny, or "unheimlich" in German, suggests a meeting between "heimlich" and "unheimlich"/ homely and unhomely / familiar and strange – meaning a place can be familiarly strange, or strange because is it unexpectedly familiar.[8] The crucial point materializes when Freud traces the numerous and complex definitions of "*heimlich*" until "*unheimlich*" surprisingly resurfaces:

> [A]mong the various shades of meaning that are recorded for the word *heimlich* there is one in which it merges with its formal antonym, *unheimlich*, so that what is called *heimlich* becomes *unheimlich*... This reminds us that this word *heimlich* is not unambiguous, but belongs to two sets of ideas, which are not mutually contradictory, but very different from each other – the one relating to what is familiar and

---

8   It is worth noting at this point the significance of Edna's words to her granddaughter, Sam, which capture the paradox of holding onto a newly alienating space as seemingly familiar but increasingly strange: "Since your grandfather passed this house seems unfamiliar. Bigger somehow. This house is the only thing left."

comfortable, the other to what is concealed and kept hidden. (Freud, 2003: 132)

The "homely" thus becomes horrifying, as a familiar domain for the dangerous and repressed, stimulating the haunting return of something that should have remained private or hidden.

The tendency of gothic horror has meant the fear of something alien coming from outside has shifted to the fear of what lies within (the home or the psyche). The doppelgänger and the split self of gothic articulate the sense of the "other" within, and repressed desire, urges and fears rising to the surface. Fear of what lies within the home (conflicts and abuses within the space that is meant to be "safe" or "homely") is clearly relevant to *Relic*. Not only do we witness Edna's violent flashes but Edna's fears of intruders coming into the home can be linked to cognitive decline, confusions over what is real, and even fear of her own family (her daughter and granddaughter) as intruders that threaten her freedom. And all three characters are violent to each other at some point. There are also the merged fears of old age that all three characters face, or will in the future face, as we do or will do, here shaped distinctively by the film's gothic tone, and by its horror genre techniques.[9]

There is in addition, though, in *Relic* a degree of developing or questioning the dualities of gothic, as it explores the shattering or blending of any clear understanding of self – of "self" and "other", of past and present. The director, James, has said that the inspiration for *Relic* came from a visit to Japan a few years before the film was made to visit her grandmother, who has Alzheimer's. And, as James expands, the first image of *Relic* grew from her grandmother's house:

---

9 Indeed, genre is key to these fine-tuned effects. We might compare the television crime film *Eizabeth is Missing* (Aisling Walsh, 2019), which conveys advancing dementia in ways that disorientate and prompt the viewer with specific clues, thus using the tools of the crime genre rather than those of horror. The merging of events and layering of perspectives to some extent also recalls B.S. Johnson's experimental, and comedic, British novel, *House Mother Normal* (1971).

> A lot of the upstairs rooms at her home were full of old junk – they
> were in essence hoarding rooms. I had this image of a hoarding room
> that just keeps going on and on. I started from there. (James, cited in
> Bell 2020)

The hoarding itself is a source for horror in *Relic*, especially as the convoluted spread mirrors the characters' confusion. It is a further reminder of time accumulating and raises questions over the sustained meaningfulness of collecting items for building a home and a sense of self. This "other" half of the house emerges in the rooms beyond locked doors and closets that stretch to form labyrinthine corridors, particularly those faced by Sam towards the end of the film, that grow and shrink unpredictably, forging dead ends and lowered ceilings that confound clarity. The shadow self also resides in the memory of the cabin where Kay's great grandfather died alone. The shocking images of a rotting corpse slipping off the bed can be attributed to Kay's repressed childhood fear that rears in nightmares. In this light, Edna's home (a beautiful fairytale cottage in the woods people dream of) becomes also the quintessential remote, creaky house inhabited by the lonely, widowed female.

The opportunity to leave this space, with its encroaching wilderness and generations of memories, is offered when Kay manages to get out to investigate the other potential space or "home", nearly half-way into the film (30–36 mins). The "retirement home" (as Kay calls it) that Kay visits in Melbourne as an initial solution is clinically stripped of excessive decor and haunting relics, in direct opposition to the family home that Edna inhabits, and Kay grew up in. However, hopes of escaping the haunted family home for a day are soon dampened on the journey there, as grey clouds hang heavily, and murmuring notes continue relentlessly on the soundtrack, approaching the urban sprawl of high-rises, viewed from the hermetically sealed, muted car. The voice-track precedes the arrival – "Now you mentioned your mother has some cognitive ... impairment..." There is a cut to the care home chessboard on the word "impairment". As the attendant and Kay walk past individuals hunched over in their chairs in their separate rooms, autonomous but in view, they pass a solemn looking man with a walker. Within earshot of the man, but oblivious of him, the attendant continues with the sales pitch, "Think of it as independent living with the edges taken off." The man stares at Kay as the woman says this and continues to watch when she turns round after they have passed. The lack of privacy and sensitivity – as residents are shown to be disconnected but not independent – speaks volumes.

Putting the film into broader context, as baby boomers (who have lived relatively independent lives) reach retirement age, there is an increased emergence of social and political concerns with how to grow old and where to live in extreme old age, or "the fourth age", as Paul Higgs and Chris Gilleard (2015) have termed the shadowy and often "othered" twilight years. While care homes have long been the locus for terror in films, novels and television dramas, the focus for that terror tends to reside in not wanting to become like the enfeebled residents. However, at this point in *Relic*, there is in addition the horror, conveyed through the combined responses of the stern male resident and the embarrassed Kay, embedded in the attendant's capitalist indifference and moral blindness – as her interest is invested solely in attaining a new resident, or recruit.

Kay is called by the woman: "Just in here." The woman, now out of focus, summons her with the big selling point: "This side of the building has ocean views." There follows the cut to the smart but most clinical looking room: the (French door style) window, and curtain, the upright blue chair, single bed, television on wall. The attendant cites the list "Handrail in every room", high toilet seat, mobility aid – which prompts Kay to praise her mother's physical abilities, "She's fit and active... not even sure she's ready for a place like this." There is a cut to close-up of Kay looking out the window, as the woman replies with a tone almost of reproach, "Well it's 5 star living". As Kay looks round then out the window, the woman's voice continues off-frame stating, "There'll be lifestyle and therapy programmes", and as she cites "disability support", there is a cut to the "sea view". We have to work to find the sea view, which is obscured by buildings, with electricity wires, cables and ugly rooves most prominently in view. The shot conveys a comedic contrast to that which is *sold*, but the moment is heart wrenching at the same time. The woman's voice continues to reel off the list of activities, but becomes faint to a distant rumble after the words "computer classes". With the cut back to the shot of Kay stood at the window, the voice trails off, and the threatening music sounds dominate, suggesting the list of activities are too inhumanly programmatic for Kay to take in, the home's sales-pitch too unsympathetic. The experience leaves Kay in tears on the way home.

It is worth pausing at this point to reflect more broadly on care homes. One of the heart-breaking aspects of the film is seeing Edna's exquisite drawings in her old sketch book. The attention to detail and to creativity can be related to the pleasures in the present associated with Edna's candle carving, where she can be slicing out great chunks of wax flesh. Embraced by the film is the joy of spontaneity, music, and loving tenderness, such as when Edna, bare foot, teaches Sam to dance. Some of the questions that might arise are how a care home or community centre might allow for long periods of contemplative creativity, where residents can be unshackled by time, without labelling the activity reductively as prescheduled "Mindful Play" within a mindless programme – driven by an ideology of keeping "busy". It is a difficult quandary because routines can also be important factors in residential homes.

In a later scene, Kay ventures into the woods to find her mother eating the family photographs – so no one can get them. Edna's fear (of something coming into the house), is a subject previously explored in James' award-winning 2017 film short Creswick (that she also co-wrote with Christian White – who co-wrote *Relic* with her), in which a father tells his daughter: "It's like someone else is living here." When Kay stops her mother from eating the photographs, Edna bites her daughter, then proceeds to then bury them, as if returning them to the ground she lives on and calls home. Her words, "I just want to go home. I just wish I could turn around and go back", are central to the whole film. The statement raises the question of what constitutes the concept of "home". Often 'home' might feel like a place, or somewhere that people or family are, or "home" might denote a sense of self – including identities that are now in the past. And this relates to Edna's question soon after this: "Where's my... Where's everyone, where is everyone?" as well as her words: "I'm losing everything Kay." Here, the notion of "losing" might include her loss of the visionary artist she once was, the friends and loved ones from her multiple younger lives and selves, especially as the memories are fading. Importantly, in a moment that marks a significant arc in Kay's journey, Kay invites her mother to move in with her, and they hug. It is a moment of togetherness. And it is a vital gesture. However, I suggest the film ends with no solution; there remains a degree of ambiguity over what will happen in terms of Edna's story, because how Kay would ever begin to navigate work and home pressures to accommodate caring for her mother is never finally resolved.

The film both confronts and elides the abiding issue that "care" still tends to remain in contemporary society the responsibility of the female. While it is possible with the three central protagonists being women to suggest that the film presents the issue as a specifically female one, the omission (or playing down) of male figures[10] might also remove some of the complexities that come with being female. Nevertheless, the breakdown of traditional family relationships is notable. Nuclear families are fragmented or conveyed only in the past, and the focus predominantly on women also allows for a simplicity, providing a spotlight on the film's central themes of aging and memory loss. The issues that come with the specifically older female living alone and the notion that "care" of all kinds is still positioned as "women's work" resound through the film, even if these factors are not explicitly foregrounded.

At the end of the film, the more monstrous horror movie mode takes over in scenes that might be read as metaphoric. A battle ensues, culminating with Kay violently, and cathartically, attacking her grasping, dying and decaying mother. But once free to escape, Kay is unable to leave Edna alone during the hardest part of her journey. Previously the voice of reason, querying her daughter's initial eagerness to move in with her gran, Kay's decision to stay with her mother at this point is crucial. After trying to flee, Sam also chooses to return. The growing mould and bruising bodies are grotesque and abject, representing a collapsing of "the border between inside and outside" (Kristeva 1982: 53),

---

10 The male appearances are brief and periphery – the law-enforcing police and the father and son next door.

rendering the film a subversive potential. Confronting the abject monstrosity of her mother's decaying body, Kay peels the hard shell of layers off, revealing a shiny breathing creature, at once hideous and beautiful. I suggest this is a subversive scene, moving beyond traditional representations of the hideous aging female, precisely because it represents a cathartic confrontation that fuses terror with emotion. As the three women lie in foetal position, the bruising mould that had been growing on Edna's body is evident and spreading on Kay, to Sam's horror. In turn it will start spreading on Sam too. The mould symbolises the threat of abandonment, as well as Edna's deterioration, so *not* leaving Edna, but being there on the journey towards and through death, even if there is the strong urge to run away, is vital to the film's end.

The reality is that the prospect of someone living alone increases with age; in Australia, over one in four people aged 65 years and over live alone (Australian Bureau of Statistics 2015). There are considerably more older women living on their own compared with older men.[11] As Robin Wood (1985: 201) argues, "One might say that the true subject of the horror genre is the struggle for recognition of all that our civilisation *r*epresses or *o*ppresses". I suggest aging, and certainly loneliness in aging, is a remaining taboo, as is the proposition that certain qualities attained through advancing years might be celebrated rather than deemed signifiers of aging badly. Many of the seemingly positive discourses surrounding "aging well" amount to the denial of aging, so that "aging well" signifies steering off traits associated with aging rather than celebrating key attributes such as attaining wrinkles, slowing down, or memory loss. However, as we age, as Segal (2014: 4) argues,

---

11   In general, older women are more likely to live on their own than older men, particularly across Europe, North America and Oceania (de Vaus and Qu 2015). As Marissa Dickins, Georgina Johnstone, Emma Renehan, Judy Lowthian and Rajna Ogrin (2022: 850) state, "In Australia, 31 per cent of older women live alone, compared with 18 per cent of older men". Adam Smith, Fran Wasoff and Lynn Jamieson (2005) report that: "Solo living is proportionately more common amongst older people. Older women are twice as likely to live alone as older men. Young men (aged 25–44) are twice as likely to live alone as young women."

we also "retain, in one manifestation or another, traces of all the selves we have been... all ages and no ages." We are old and as a child at the same time. This amounts to "complex layerings of identity" (Segal 2014: 4) unique to aging and uniquely forged by it.

While a key part of the horror in *Relic* is that dementia can be inherited, the film to some extent also offers a move on from concepts related to "decline" and "degeneration", often associated with dementia. I use the term "regeneration" in the title of this chapter – due to a refreshing sense of understanding and confrontation the film encourages, raising questions about how quality of life can be improved in old age or how older people can feel better integrated. The film unites three generations of women whose experiences and emotions merge. It is not only about the fear of how a person feels when a loved one begins to feel losses, but also about experiencing these emotionally ourselves. James (cited in Kelley 2020) has said "if [the film] helps someone process the experience in a new way or helps them conquer that fear, that would be pretty amazing." The final scare of *Relic* is that what is afflicting some now will affect others into the future. The film encourages caring and confronting rather than retreating. It does not provide neat solutions and remains ambivalent about the processes involved in navigating work and home pressures to take care of elderly relatives, but there is plenty for contemplation and debate. It taps into the conflicting emotions that concern most families, as a daughter or son who was once cared for must reverse roles. It resonates with the worry we have about support for the elderly, the practicalities for achieving good care, and keeping well ourselves in the process – the fears of the mistakes we are bound to make, and others might in turn make with us.

The care home in *Relic* insists it allows "independence", but the film encourages us to accept *dependence* (possibly one of the hardest aspects for contemporary populations to accept) as a part of the human condition. As Sally Chivers and Ulla Kriebernegg (2017: 17) observe:

> While people adamantly desire to age well at home, without making the big move to render their latter years more manageable, and policy makers play to that desire, apparently buoyed by how it offers them

an opportunity to download the costs of care onto the family unit, the fact remains that many contemporary senior citizens will require institutional care, and some might even choose it.

As humans age, and the future promises far less time than the past, individual successes often become less meaningful. This philosophy might act as a reminder of the *vanitas* image explored near the beginning of this chapter. Stuart Hall (cited in Segal 2014: 275) reportedly claimed that as he got older he believed "less and less in the language of the independent self, personal achievement, the autonomy of the individual", clarifying "we are never self-sustaining but constituted by others who are different from us". This emphasis on the collective locates the concept of "home" somewhere between a place called "home" and that place we feel at home – safe but attached to the world. Most of the commercially driven positivity surrounding aging is in real terms the negation of aging, but there is so much in aging that we might embrace. Timetabling tends to permeate our lives from the nursery through to the end of our working adult lives. Extreme old age can be a time to explore new selves and consciousnesses. And perhaps it is human connection (across generations), with equally the possibility of creative contemplation, laughter, music, opportunity, privacy, spontaneity, and unaudited solitude when needed, that we might try to focus on with regards to thinking meaningfully about the concept of what constitutes a good "home" and "proper care" – or what models of "better" care might consist of.

Author Bio

Professor Laura Hubner is author of the monographs *Fairytale and Gothic Horror: Uncanny Transformations in Film* and *The Films of Ingmar Bergman: Illusions of Light and Darkness*. She is editor of *Valuing Films: Shifting Perceptions of Worth*, and co-editor of *The Zombie Renaissance in Popular Culture* and *Framing Film: Cinema and the Visual Arts*. Currently Professor of Film and Media at the University of Winchester, UK, she was recently Guest Speaker for the 1000th Edition of BBC Radio 4's *In Our Time* on Bergman's

The Seventh Seal, and her next monograph on Bergman launches the book series she is editing, *Iconic Movie Images*.

Works Cited

Australian Bureau of Statistics (2015) Household and Family Projections, Australia, 2011 to 2036. Canberra: Australian Bureau of Statistics.

Barthes, Roland (1982): Camera Lucida: Reflections on Photography, translated by R. Howard, New York: Hill and Wang.

Bell, James (2020): "'There's heartbreak in someone losing themselves': Relic director Natalie Erika James on her love of gothic and Asian horror." In: Sight and Sound, October 28, https://www.bfi.org.uk/sight-and-sound/interviews/natalie-erika-james-relic-influences-gothic-asian-horror [accessed August 1 2022].

Chivers, Sally/Kriebernegg, Ulla, (2017): "Introduction." In: Sally Chivers/Ulla Kriebernegg (eds.), Care Home Stories: Aging, Disability, and Long-Term Residential Care, Aging Studies Volume XIV, Bielefeld: transcript, pp. 17–26.

Creed, Barbara (1993): The Monstrous-Feminine: Film, Feminism, Psychoanalysis, London: Routledge.

de Vaus, David and Qu, Lixia (2015): Living Alone and Personal Wellbeing, Australian Family Trend 10, Melbourne: Australian Institute of Family Studies.

Dickins Marissa/Johnstone Georgina/Renehan Emma/Lowthian Judy/Ogrin Rajna (2022). "The Barriers and Enablers to Service Access for Older Women Living Alone in Australia." In: Ageing and Society 42, pp. 849–867.

Eizabeth is Missing (Aisling Walsh, 2019)

Freud, Sigmund (2003): "The Uncanny" (1919). In: The Uncanny, translated by D. McLintock, London: Penguin Classics, pp. 123–162.

Higgs, Paul and Gilleard, Chris (2015): Rethinking Old Age: Theorising the Fourth Age, London and New York: Palgrave Macmillan.

Johnson, B.S. (1971): House Mother Normal.

Kelley, Sonaiya (2020): "Emily Mortimer explains the 'extraordinary and bizarre' ending of 'Relic.'" In: Los Angeles Times July 10, https://www.latimes.com/entertainment-arts/movies/story/2020-07-10/relic-ending-explained-emily-mortimer [accessed August 15 2022].

Kermode, Mark (2020): "Relic review – heartbreaking horror about Alzheimer's." In: The Guardian Sunday November 1, https://www.theguardian.com/film/2020/nov/01/relic-review-natalie-erika-james-emily-mortimer-alzheimers-horror [accessed August 1 2022].

Kristeva, Julia (1982): Powers of Horror: An Essay on Abjection, translated by Leon S. Roudiez, New York and Chichester, West Sussex: Columbia University Press.

Matheson Sue (2019): "'More like music': Aging, Abjection and Dementia at the Overlook Hotel". In: Cynthia J. Miller/A. Bowdoin Van Riper (eds.), Elder Horror: Essays on Film's Frightening Images of Aging, Jefferson, North Carolina: McFarland and Company, Inc.

Relic (Natalie Erika James, 2020)

Relic entry on the International Movies Database https://www.imdb.com/title/tt9072352/ [accessed August 16 2022].

Segal, Lynne (2014): Out of Time: The Pleasures and Perils of Ageing, London, New York: Verso.

Smith, Adam/Wasoff, Fran/Jamieson, Lynn (2005): *Solo Living Across the Adult Lifecourse*, Edinburgh, Research Briefing 20, Centre for Research on Families and Relationships, https://era.ed.ac.uk/bitstream/handle/1842/2822/rb20.pdf;jsessionid=8F83A095410D69B2B796425F9CBD193B?sequence=1 via: https://www.crfr.ac.uk [accessed August 18 2022].

The Visit (M. Night Shyamalan, 2015)

Whatever Happened to Baby Jane (Robert Aldrich, 1962)

Wood, Robin (1985): "An Introduction to the American Horror Film." In: Bill Nichols (ed.), Movies and Methods Volume II: An Anthology, Berkeley, Los Angeles, London: University of California Press, pp. 195–220.